Oh No!
I Have Cancer,
Now What?

by

Marilyn Bray

Book design by Ben Cornatzer, www.outtamymind.net

A special thank you to my brother Frank for his unconditional love, for understanding that Sis could not be with him as much, and for embracing his time with Dee. We both were blessed to have Dee, his caregiver, to support us.

Dedicated to Nicole, Anna, Rosemary, June, Candy, Pat, Mary Louise, Marianne, and Caryn who were the strength of my support team.

Thank you to Vicki who convinced me to write my story after I was determined not to do it. Vicki lost her mother to cancer.

To everyone who crossed my path and offered any kindness during my journey with breast cancer, I am deeply grateful. Without you, my journey would have been quite different.

"… Your journey has presented
so many challenges
and yet you faced each one with
strength, beauty, and grace.
… May you continue to fight
the good fight and enjoy
the miracles along the way.
All our love!"

— family friends at the beach (OBX)

Table of Contents

Foreword
9

Imaging and Identification of Malignant Tumors
11

Surgery
23

Chemo or Not
33

Radiation Next
74

Recovery
87

Lessons Learned
97

Acknowledgements
99

Foreword

This book is written from the heart by a remarkable woman and friend who has shown strength, selflessness, as well as compassion by wanting to use her personal story to guide other patients and their families. Her emotions are raw and honest.

Marilyn and I met in a dimly lit ultrasound room of the diagnostic breast cancer center in which I work during one of her most vulnerable moments. Minutes before, the 3D mammogram images before my eyes showed me that she likely had breast cancer, as demonstrated by the presence of a new, irregular mass. Despite this unfamiliar reality, Marilyn and I connected professionally in a patient-doctor relationship as she guided our conversation with an array of thoughtful questions regarding her possible diagnosis. Even though Marilyn may have felt overwhelmed as I spoke regarding the need to do a breast biopsy, her calm, approachable, yet inquisitive manner allowed me to address her questions and concerns easily.

As a physician, one of the biggest privileges I have experienced is the trust and knowledge shared between two humans. Even after years, delivering the news to a person that they need a biopsy and may have breast cancer still isn't easy. I consider myself fortunate to be a part of my patients' lives, and they continue to teach me how to serve them better. Marilyn exemplifies this; she encourages and strengthens me as a radiologist. Her optimism is empowering.

In reading Marilyn's book, it's important to remember that everyone's cancer mindset will be different. Regardless, she shares how she herself confronts and battles her life-changing diagnosis with endless fortitude, optimism, and hope. This is one patient's perspective, and this book is not intended to pave the path for anyone else's journey. It is a true story of how one woman applied her intelligence, embraced her beloved brother and friends, and took advantage of all available resources to cope. I hope that this book will serve to provide a strongly optimistic perspective and inspire each of you to remain positive throughout your or your loved one's journey. If it does, then I know it will have achieved its desired intention.

Nicole Kelleher, M.D., M.S.

Favorite websites:

Breastcancer.org
www.breastcancer.org

American Cancer Society
www.cancer.org

National Breast Cancer Foundation
www.nationalbreastcancer.org

Additional Sites:

National Cancer Institute
www.cancer.gov

Virginia Breast Cancer Foundation
www.vbcf.org

Imaging and Identification of Malignant Tumors

"I am going to be honest with you. I think you have breast cancer." I am calm on the outside, but my mind is trying to gather my thoughts. I live with my 54-year-old brother, Frank, who has Down Syndrome. I am his legal guardian and full-time caregiver. We have no other family. This diagnosis is about to change life in some way for both of us.

August 23

I return for an ultrasound of my breast two weeks after my annual mammogram. I have been called back in previous years and am not concerned at this point. The technician zooms in on one area. She seems to focus on one spot. As I watch the screen, I am suspicious of a problem here. She completes the ultrasound and leaves to get the radiologist. Immediately, I suspect something is not good. As the radiologist is doing the ultrasound on my breast, it is obvious to me that the "black blob" on the screen is something of significance.

I ask her what she thinks it might be. Her answer is not what I want to hear. "I am going to be honest with you. I think you have breast cancer." I ask how often she is correct in her predictions. She says 97%. It gets my attention. For her to give me a preliminary diagnosis and be this confident with it, I realize I am beginning an unknown journey. I ask if my many years of taking hormone replacement medications caused my cancer. She tells me the meds may have advanced it but not caused it. The number one reason is being a woman over 50. Even though I am at a low risk for breast cancer, it has appeared. I am grateful for the radiologist's honesty and willingness to share her thinking. She is informative and compassionate and gives me all the time I need. As we discuss it, she says it probably means lumpectomy and radiation. She tells me that I can get through it. The next step will be an ultrasound core biopsy of this tumor. With the information I received, I am thinking that survival issues are off the table. I do not need to spend time spinning with the possibilities. Yes, it is difficult to not go there, especially with my guardianship of Frank and not having a clear direction of what might happen to him should I die first. As I leave the radiology area, I am thankful the tumor was identified and will be treated. I am most grateful for my discussion with the radiologist. She has set the tone for my journey. Now I need to own it. It will take time for me to absorb this diagnosis.

After scheduling an appointment for the biopsy, I walk to my car, call Anna, and then drive home to begin my research. I know NOTHING about breast cancer.

Happy Birthday to me! I think I will remember this birthday forever. It certainly is not on my list of ways to celebrate. I am glad I celebrated two days ago at the beach.

I am stunned and overwhelmed. My life changed instantly with this preliminary diagnosis. It is consuming my thinking. Where do I begin? I listened intently to the radiologist who has given me direction and hope for this journey. Now I have choices to make. I can panic and not trust what she shared, or I can focus only on what she is telling me and take it one step at a time.

I choose to trust the radiologist who identifies breast cancer issues daily. I know it will be difficult to keep me narrowly focused and not let my mind wander to the what ifs. I begin by googling "ultrasound core biopsy." I read information on multiple sights. I want to know how the lump will be biopsied. It is important to me to understand all procedures I will undergo. I am convinced that knowledge is power. If I understand, my stress will not become a huge problem and take me down. It will empower me to be more comfortable in discussions with the medical professionals.

I plan to be a participant in my care and not a reactor. I am a questioner and want to understand everything about my health. I approach this journey unlike other serious medical concerns my family or I have experienced in the past.

I read about the types of breast cancer, stages, treatments, prognosis, and recurrence rates for each stage. I remember the radiologist telling me the tumor is small. How does size impact my treatment? After hours of reading and rereading over several days, I narrow my sources to the websites that give me the clarity and depth I want. I want information that is factual, explains well, and helps me understand. I treat this learning process as an academic journey. I am mentally exhausted from my research and knowing I have a cancer journey in front of me. There are many unknowns at this point. It seems like I am taking a cram course, and time is running out. I need a break.

Whenever stressed, I try to pull back and do something to restore my balance. I begin taking more long walks to get away from it. I listen to music or a podcast. I live in a community with ample walking trails and enjoy frequent walks. Being outdoors is a stress reliever for me. It also keeps me off the computer and wanting to investigate more. Additionally, I talk to Marianne, a neighbor. She listens and assures me that she will be there throughout this journey.

I am more introverted than extroverted. I enjoy my alone time and prefer small groups over crowds. I am not one to share my inner thoughts other than with close friends. Quickly, I am realizing that I may need to reach out more than I ever have. I am extremely independent and recognize

I may need to step out of my comfort zone to be open to all support.

My worries are more about Frank than my cancer. How will I be able to handle it all? How do I protect him? If he needs to know later, what do I say so he can understand and know that I will be okay? What do I need to do to have everything for him should my prognosis become more serious? I am a planner and always have a backup plan. It is one way of keeping me grounded. I keep a three-ring binder with everything one needs to know about Frank in case something happens to me. Although I do not see survival being an issue, I see a wakeup call to update his binder and decide about his future guardian.

To be proactive, I call Frank's caregiver and ask if she can come once a week. We have no regular schedule with Dee. It is an "as needed" basis. I want to have support in place to take some pressure off me. I may be at home but will need breaks from being responsible for his total care. Frank had been independent until two years ago. He had a near-death experience that would take him 12–14 months to recover and a cervical fusion before he fully got through that recovery. It has impacted his ability to think. He has increasing familial tremors which are unrelated to Down Syndrome. Our mother had them, too. He struggles with writing which is his most important activity. He wants me to write for him when his

Getting good healthcare is a partnership between the patient and medical community. It requires effort.

special TV programs come on. He struggles with eating independently. He cannot get the fork to his mouth because of his tremors and lack of strength from his health issues. I have changed menus to having foods that he can "stab" as he tells me. With other foods, he needs assistance. The large, weighted silverware no longer solves his shakiness.

The internet is loaded with personal stories of people dealing with breast cancer. I am making a conscious decision to avoid them. Too many of them are not fact-based and may not relate to my specific diagnosis. We all are different. I need to understand the medical aspects of my preliminary diagnosis and the care for it. I always find that when I understand, I am calmer and have easier recoveries. It is my goal for this journey.

I am on overload. I need some time to absorb the magnitude of this diagnosis and get a plan for attacking it. Never did I think I would have a cancer diagnosis. I identify close friends whom I want to know. I talk with my pastor and request that he keep it confidential until I have reached my friends. I do not want them to hear it from someone else. The responses are similar. My friends are stunned, concerned for me, and offer support throughout the months ahead. I assure them I will let them know when I need help.

My biggest concern is going to church and being bombarded with comments. It is one reason I am keeping a tighter control on who knows at this point. I need time. When I leave home, I do not want "cancer" in my face all day. A few years ago, a colleague was diagnosed with her second event with breast cancer. I asked her why she chose to keep it quiet and not share. Her comment hit home with me. "I do not need to be reminded of my cancer every time I see someone at work. This is the one place where I can get away from it. The intentions are good, but it is too hard for me."

September 1
When I return for this appointment, I tell the technician that I have some questions for the radiologist. When she arrives, she sits on the exam table next to me and welcomes my

questions. My mind is full of so many thoughts. She spends considerable time helping me understand the preliminary diagnosis and putting it into context. I learn that there is always the possibility of micrometastases in the lymph nodes even though my nodes appear to be clear. It means there could be micro cancer cells found during surgery. The node is sliced many times to find them. They are a concern but do not carry the same significance as finding tumors in the lymph nodes. What I most appreciate is the radiologist's willingness to answer anything and everything I ask. Her answers reinforce what I have read. This discussion gives me a huge level of support and clarity. Now I need to focus on what she shared and not let my mind run in crazy directions. This process is requiring me to be highly disciplined in my thinking. It is an effort.

I watch the ultrasound core biopsy and am intrigued. There are no surprises since the radiologist explained it, and I am informed from my reading. There is no discomfort. It is obvious to me that fear and the unknown can drive pain for many patients. I know what will be done and trust this physician. I cannot control the diagnosis or procedures. I can choose how I respond to them. I ask the radiologist what she is thinking. She suspects I have invasive ductal carcinoma and shares information about it. After the biopsy, there is a follow-up mammogram. The radiologist returns, asks me to come to her office, and shows me another tumor behind the one she biopsied. It was not visible until now. I certainly did not see this one coming or think about the possibility. She gives me a choice to return later for a second biopsy or have it done now. I am appreciative of her willingness to do it immediately. After the second biopsy is taken, she tells me this one looks different. Of course, I begin questioning the implications of having different cancers and how it might impact treatment. Both tumors are in the same quadrant which is positive. Both tumors are small which is another positive. The radiologist continues to anticipate I will have a lumpectomy and radiation. My mind is muddled after this second biopsy. I am not sure I am understanding all of it.

I will return to receive the pathology results and then move to the surgeon. I now will need an MRI for both breasts. The surgeon will be the one to order it.

The radiologist gives me her business card with her email and cell phone. She encourages me to contact her if I have questions anytime during my journey. She tells me that each physician I encounter will be on my team. The teams meet weekly to discuss the individual cases. She always will be on my team. I had no idea a radiologist would continue care once I leave imaging. It is obvious that she is available to support me through this journey, not only today. Never have I experienced this level of support from a physician who is not a family physician. It is different. It is real. I need to pay attention to having this resource when I have concerns. I leave the hospital with my mind racing again. Every time I think I am a step closer to surgery, something else happens. I am wondering when I will be done with the imaging. More questions are flooding my thinking.

I am noticing a huge sense of community in those who treat patients for breast cancer. I have dealt with a physician and support staff in the imaging unit. It is different from what I typically experience in the medical world. I certainly would never choose cancer or to be in this position. However, the care has been compassionate, encouraging, and supportive. I have been asked by support staff where I am getting my questions. In response, I ask what they typically see. I understand most patients are angry, grieving, and crying. I have not dealt with those emotions, probably because of this radiologist's approach and survival not seeming to be an issue at this point. I generally am positive in my outlook. I am educating myself after each visit and trying not to look too far ahead. I want to be a participant in my health care. I am convinced that my learning about the procedure today made it easier for me to ask questions, participate in a discussion with the radiologist, and learn about my cancer.

I am more focused on getting the best physicians for me, understanding everything about my cancer, and preparing for the next step. The radiologist is a wealth of knowledge and extremely supportive. If she does not have the answer, she tells me my surgeon will be able to respond better. Already, she is changing my narrow perception of the role of a radiologist. The open communications are helping me stay balanced and not panic. It is clear to me that if I do my part in trying to understand and talk openly with the physician, I have a stronger chance of getting through this journey well. I am not one to react out of fear. I grew up with fear and finally learned to conquer it. For me, fear can come with the unknown. It is why I want to educate myself and avoid the unknown.

I am not scared but exhausted. I am spending hours on the laptop. I am thinking about cancer every waking moment. Sometimes the information is not clear to me. There are too many new terms. I send an email to the radiologist and ask for clarification. Her response began, "I am so glad you reached out to me." They are powerful words of support to someone scrambling to figure out this breast cancer world. It helped that I did not have to wait until my next office visit to get answers. I did not have to stress about it after she provided clarity. I am not one to overly stress about a diagnosis or procedures. I do stress with wait time in getting answers. She took that stress away from me.

I said to Anna, who has known me for many years, "I seem unusually calm." She agreed and said she was totally surprised. I honestly attribute it to the initial communications with this compassionate radiologist and her availability to answer questions. One of her statements to me was, "Breast cancer is an emotional and physical challenge. You are strong both emotionally and physically and will do well.' She continues to set a positive tone for my health journey. Cancer is a life changer. I hung on every word the radiologist said at each visit. The power of her words gives me strength, direction, a sense of calmness, and a safety net. Now I must own it and do my part.

I have been able to continue living as if there is no cancer. I feel good. Frank and I are maintaining our routine. The only differences are less time at the beach and my thinking about cancer. We are fortunate to have access to a family beach house in the Outer Banks. We generally spend most weeks there in the fall. The beach is my happy place.

I hold on to two beliefs. Cancer will not define me. I will continue living my life and slow down or stop when needed. I want Frank to live his life and not take on my cancer issues. I see no reason to tell him at this point. I know it will be hard on him.

A few days later, I drive to the Williamsburg Outlets. I had pre-planned a shopping trip. It is a beautiful day. I decide to sit on a bench and make some phone calls. I call Rosemary, a friend and former colleague, to get someone's cell phone number. Then I call June and Candy. June and I were colleagues. Candy and I knew each other through our church. Both had breast cancer recently. I want to know which physicians they chose and how it worked for them. I ask about the type of cancer, lymph node involvement, surgery, problems encountered, and treatment options. Already I am armed with information from other professionals and what I read on the internet about each surgeon. I talked with my family physician. Additionally, I reviewed the Richmond Magazine Top Docs issues for the past three years. The physicians are rated by their peers. I am not looking to make a quick decision. I only want to gather more information. I need to apply what I am learning to what will work for me. At this point I have a short list of physicians who may be good for me. June and Candy are incredible in sharing their personal stories and offering support beyond today. Their stories are not the same. They used different physicians and hospitals. One had an easy path; the other one encountered some difficulties. Within an hour, it becomes clear to me who my choices will be. I did not expect clarity so soon. I am relieved to have these decisions made. I can take this stress off my plate. These decisions are huge. They probably are the most important decisions I will make. Trusting my physicians will be critical in my care. I do not want to be in a position of second guessing myself.

I want a surgeon who spends a high percentage of his/her time with breast cancer patients and is recognized for knowledge, surgical skills, and guiding patients through the decision-making process. I want a medical oncologist who works with many breast cancer patients and who will work with me on whatever odd things might happen. I am healthy but am called an outlier by my family physician. Odd medical situations occur with me. Because I look healthy, some physicians overlook my concerns.

Five years ago, I had a serious issue with my lower leg after a major back surgery. It was unlike any symptom I have ever experienced. On my first day home, I was walking in the driveway. Each time I put weight on that leg, I got excruciating pain in my calf. When my weight shifted, there was no pain. I was convinced it was unrelated to the back. The neurosurgeon did not believe me. He refused to consider other possibilities even though I was greatly limited and dealing with intense pain. He thought it was a recovery concern with my back surgery and would take time to heal. Weeks later, I decided to see a vascular surgeon and could not get in for two months with the one I wanted. I took first available. It was one of the worst mistakes I have made in my years of health care. On my fourth visit, he advocated for surgery on both legs, even though the horrific symptoms involved only one leg. He obviously was not hearing me. Nine months after my back surgery, a serious diagnosis was made by a radiology interventionalist. I had a completely blocked artery from genetic cholesterol in my lower leg and could have lost my foot. Since I never had any cholesterol concerns in prior years, this information surprised everyone. Obviously, I had never been tested for genetic cholesterol. It was not part of the standard blood tests. Because I was months past my surgery date, it was too late to have a stent placed in the artery. The risk of throwing a clot that could kill me was high. However, I could regain function by pushing through the pain and walking daily. It was music to my ears when this radiologist offered hope and concrete suggestions. I had been walking daily since it occurred. It took me twice as long to walk and with tears many times. Walking with a purpose would strengthen the collateral arteries so they would take over and allow me to continue with what I want to do. This experience magnified my need to be where these odd situations are not unusual. I want to know I will be heard if something odd occurs.

I am choosing to use services at two hospitals. It is a personal choice and one that each individual needs to make based on their own needs. It is not what most patients choose. I have been assured that all care will be coordinated between these providers. I prefer to stay close to home if I am comfortable with the services offered. I will have surgery, imaging, and radiation at my community hospital. I am choosing a teaching hospital for the medical oncology. Now that I have selected physicians for surgery, medical oncology, and radiation oncology, I need a plan for approaching the upcoming months.

At this point, I am thinking only about lumpectomy and radiation. I honestly believe I can handle it without much change at home. I have endured multiple surgeries and always done well. I am more concerned about interference with other plans for the holidays and attending the UVA men's basketball games. The sooner I get through it, the better.

September 7
Anna and I meet with the radiologist and the nurse navigator for the breast cancer unit. I ask Anna to take notes and to feel free to ask questions. At this meeting, I receive my pathology results. I have invasive ductal carcinoma and invasive lobular carcinoma in the same breast and in the same quadrant. The hormone receptor results work in my favor with one exception. The HER2 is equivocal which means further testing needs to be done. The FISH test will be run to get clarification on it. At this point, I have stage 1 early breast cancer. I keep in mind that surgery may reveal micrometastases in the lymph nodes. After responding to questions, the radiologist leaves. The nurse navigator explains her role and provides a resource manual. She, too, is available for any questions I may have during this journey.

I do find this meeting frustrating because the room is too crowded for four people. The radiologist has to stand. It is difficult for me to focus since we are on top of each other. I am glad Anna is taking notes, so I can clarify later. It is the first time that too much is coming at me too fast. I hear but am not absorbing all of it. I truly attribute it to my discomfort with the close quarters and not the information shared.

I am relieved to have completed the procedures in radiology and know that I will see a surgeon soon. However, it feels as if the rug is being pulled out from me. I want to get out of radiology but have found a comfort zone with the personnel here.

I am a strong advocate for patient portals. I use my portal at the hospital and find all radiology reports. It is helpful for me to read them again. If I do not understand something, I can ask the physician at my next appointment or send an email to the radiologist.

I also keep a medical journal for my brother and me. I document every medical visit. When concerns arise. I write them down for the next visit. For me, once I have it on paper, I do not need to keep thinking about it. Then two days preceding my appointment, I read my notes and prepare for the visit. I learned this tactic to maximize my appointment and relieve stress.

I have a two-week planned trip to South Dakota coming soon. I inquired about my taking the trip or should I postpone it. The radiologist said it is important that I take the trip and continue enjoying my activities. It will not impact my cancer. I have enough experience to understand the process of getting to surgery can take weeks. It helps me justify following through with this trip. I also know I truly need to do something different. The timing of the trip is perfect for me.

Frank is thrilled I am leaving. He loves being with the caregiver and doing new activities. It is his vacation, too. While gone, I post a picture on Facebook and call it, "Good times in the Badlands." Dee, in return, posts a picture with Frank, neighbors, and herself. She titles it, "Good times in Woodlake." Frank's smile is huge! I love seeing him having so much fun, especially with new situations for him.

The trip is a wonderful get away from the cancer world. For the first two days, I am preoccupied with cancer. I often interject questions and comments with my friend. By the third day, I shift gears and push it to the back of my mind. I think about it, but have no need to talk about it, probably because of many new experiences. It surprises both my friend and me. I strongly recommend that newly diagnosed cancer patients continue living and take these mental health breaks. They are important, especially since a long journey awaits.

Surgery

I am entering the next chapter of this journey
and have more preparation to do. I begin research-
ing lumpectomies versus mastectomies. I want to
know what the data show about recurrence with
each one. I also research reconstructive surgery in
case I might choose a mastectomy.

September 19

The surgeon answers my questions. Discussions
are brief since we lack all information. She does
inform me that the FISH, done to clarify the
HER2 on tumors in my left breast, is negative.
The result works to my benefit. The surgeon
orders an MRI because of the multiple tumors
and two different cancers and gives me a follow-
up appointment. Anna accompanies me and takes
notes. She kindly has offered to be with me
at all key appointments. I am grateful to have
her presence. I know that I may not remember
everything.

The surgeon's assistant warns me there may be a
wait to have an MRI. When she calls, there is
a cancellation for one in two days. I am relieved.
Later I learn my insurance company will not

approve it without a three-day notice. The assistant is not able to get it approved and suggests I might want to make a call. Obviously, it will get approved at some point. I call the insurance company and get the same answer. I hang up, call again, and get a different agent. This agent's response is, "When a physician places a request for a quick turnaround, our job is to help you and get it through." Sometimes rules are not as rigid as they appear. It seems to depend on the how good the agent is with customer service and how I present the issue. When a barrier appears and makes no sense to me, I try to find a way to go around it. I do not want to have an unnecessary delay. I want to have this MRI and move on to surgery.

September 21
I have the breast MRI. Several hours later as I am driving to the Outer Banks, the surgeon calls about a concern in the other breast. She will schedule me for an MRI guided biopsy. I am not sure how to respond. What else will they find? I ask her if an additional tumor will decrease my odds of getting through this journey? She says no. I ask if it will change the surgery. She again says no. It has raised my concerns. I call Anna and ask if she is surprised. She has known me for years and is well versed with my medical history. She responds, "No, because you are an outlier." Once again, I see more odd situations with my medical world.

I am appreciative of having the MRI. Otherwise, I may have faced a more serious cancer in a few years since it did not appear on the mammogram. Not everyone is offered the MRI because of their individual situation, and not every surgeon sees the need for it. I read about this procedure for the biopsy, so I know what is coming.

Rosemary stops by on her way home from work. We freely chat, and she offers a prayer as she departs. She has kept up with my journey and will text, call, or visit before each procedure or appointment. We laugh and enjoy our time together. She always is thoughtful, encouraging, and supportive in multiple ways. Her friendship has offered me a strong lifeline.

September 26
I meet with the radiologist, have the MRI guided biopsy explained to me, and sign more consent forms. There is ample time for questions. I know what to expect but cannot observe this one because of my positioning. My challenge is being still for a long length of time. Having an MRI of any kind is one of my least favorite tests. I lie there thinking that I have cancer, and it will take forever to get to surgery. It has been a month since my diagnosis, and I continue to need more procedures. I want this cancer out of my body. Even though I understand it probably took years to develop, I want immediate action.

I qualified for genetic testing at my surgical appointment and return for an appointment with the nurse practitioner. She explains the types of cancer to be considered, why we are doing it, and how it is done. This test is optional. More forms are signed. I return later for the results. Fortunately, I have no genetic concerns in the results.

This cancer journey is a mind exercise. I daily work at staying focused on learning and preparing for the next step. Many times, I find myself stopping other thoughts that want to get in the way. Staying positive is a MUST!

September 28
I meet with the surgeon to discuss the MRI results and surgery for breast cancer. She has a draft of the tumor pathology in the other breast. It appears to be lobular cancer. It has not been confirmed. She reviews my surgical options. I am most interested in the data about results for each option. Discussions are longer and with more details. The surgeon recommends the lumpectomies because the data does not support an outcome difference by choosing mastectomies. Since I am not one to worry excessively, I want the least invasive surgery. I also know that if I choose mastectomies, I most likely will want reconstructive surgery. It is an elective surgery with a difficult recovery and risk of complications. The surgeon shows me exercises for arm movement to begin after surgery. We also discuss data about recurrence and survival. I inquire about treatment for a recurrence. She emphasizes it does not necessarily mean I would need a mastectomy. I am scheduled

for surgery on October 12th. The surgeon requests her assistant to make appointments for me to see the medical and radiation oncologists soon after surgery. Treatment should begin within a month. I leave there thinking I may be able to complete this journey by early January if radiation is the only recommendation. I am feeling good.

Thus far, friends have not noticed any changes in me. I appear to be the same as ever. I generally am calm on the outside. The changes so far are within me with my thinking about cancer most of the day. Even though all seems doable so far, I am cognizant of other possibilities appearing. I am not sure when I will know all I need to know.

October 5
I decide to tell Frank I have breast cancer. I want him to hear it from me and not someone else during a conversation. He will need time to process it. He seems to listen to most everything going on with me. We are having dinner. He is alert and having fun teasing me. I tell him I have a lump in my breast, and it needs to come out. I add that our mother had a lump removed and did well. I know I will do well, too. He rests his head in his hands and tells me to take it out of his head. He does not like to hear bad news. He is visibly concerned. I reassure him that Dee will be with him, and I will come home that night. I refer to times that I have needed his help after orthopedic surgeries. I remind him he may have to help me. I continue telling him I will be okay. Frank increases his self-talking when he is alone. It is his way of understanding. It also gives me more insight into his concerns.

The next day, I can see his anxiety is up. We sit and chat. I reassure him that I am going to "kick this cancer out of my body." I know I will be okay, but it will take time. Again, he tells me to take it out of his head. He does not want to hear the word "cancer." I have learned with Frank that less is more. Give the minimum and leave it alone.

We serve dinner at church on Wednesday evenings. I notice Frank is getting phone numbers of people he does not know. I ask about it. He tells me he needs it "just in case you be up there with Mom and the boys (our two older deceased brothers)." I am seeing that he is going to need lots of reassurance. We are in uncharted territory. His security is being threatened.

I find friends and ask them to focus on one comment to Frank, that Sis will be okay. He will need to hear it over and over. I have not sat him down and talked about what will happen should I die before him. He will obsess at the thought of it. Hopefully, I will be here for him always. However, he does need more support.

I decide to get counseling for Frank. I want to be proactive and give him someone with whom to talk freely. Sometimes, he will hold back with me if he thinks it will be upsetting. I also want an extra set of eyes on him. I know I will be preoccupied and not as observant during this journey.

I begin sharing my medical status more openly with others and release my pastor to share as well. I am more grounded and think I can handle it. It takes time to own a cancer diagnosis. The responses are overwhelming. I am thinking I am okay if the plan for surgery and radiation remain the same. Thus far, we are plugging along as we always do. When Dee is here with Frank, she always helps me, too.

It is interesting to me to see how others respond to hearing I have cancer. Most jump in with support. A few do not know what to say and avoid mentioning it. I take the lead in making everyone comfortable. It is a fact of life. I am not embarrassed by it. I do not feel the need to be secretive. I only request that I have my space when needed. My closest friends, without my saying anything, know to keep life normal and keep me going with what I love about life. They are there when I may stumble.

I am approached by a staff member at church who wants me to join the breast cancer support group there. I thank her and share that I am way ahead. I created my support group quickly with friends a month ago. It includes friends who have dealt with breast cancer, friends from church, and others whom I value. Additionally, because of full-time caregiving responsibilities, my time away from home is limited. I do not need to take on something that duplicates or does not fit my needs. I must be selective with my time.

I meet Megan for lunch. I taught Megan's children years ago. Immediately, she says, "Marilyn, you know how independent you are. You will need to allow support." She continues. I hold up my hand, stop her, and assure her that decision has been made. I keep a list on my phone of friends who offer to help. The inconvenience of surgery is not new to me. However, with cancer, I honestly do not know how I will respond. I am focused on taking it one day at a time and not looking too far ahead. I have endured many surgeries but have never approached any of them as I am doing this time.

I am missing my extended time at the beach. Instead of taking 2–3 weeks with each visit, I am adjusting to long weekends because of the numerous medical appointments. I know I need to find ways to get there. Frank and I go there for three nights. It gives me a chance to let my beach friends know that I may not return for a few months. There are too many unknowns. I am overwhelmed. They reach out in ways I never would have anticipated. I have focused on Frank for years and watched so much good come to him. It is odd for me to be in this situation where the focus is on me. Additionally, a total stranger reached out to me at a store. She overheard me mention I had breast cancer. She gave me a small token with the word "healing" on it and wished me well. I left the beach to come home and felt somewhat emotional about the kindnesses I experienced on this trip.

Each time Frank sees someone he knows, he expresses his concern about what might happen to him if I "go up above." I ask all friends to tell him repeatedly that "Sis will get well. It will take time." Although I am telling him I will be okay, he is unsure. It is a heartbreaker to watch him go through it.

Beyond my two brief conversations with Frank about cancer, I have avoided mentioning it in our home or in front of him elsewhere. I am trying to keep him out of it as best possible. At times, I take my phone outside to have conversations about my health.

October 11
Pre-op is scheduled at the last minute by the hospital. I was called two days ago. Fortunately, I took myself off aspirin a week ago. I learned it from prior experiences. Had I not made that change, my surgery would have been postponed. I would not have been happy. The exam is brief since the surgeon has most of the needed information. Surgery is set for tomorrow morning.

I tell Anna that I will drive myself to the hospital and get my car later. It will be a long day. There is little she can do. I prefer that she not come until an hour or so before the surgery ends. I want her available to chat with the surgeon. Upon arrival, I will have two procedures prior to surgery. I will be busy and am not one to want lots of commotion. I like a calm environment. I also anticipate there will be little, if any, downtime. Anna knows me well enough to know that I am okay.

I have recently discovered that a close friend is an alcoholic. I am stunned and saddened. I have observed strange behaviors with her in recent years but had not connected the dots. I have shifted my energies in recent days from cancer to reading about alcoholism. After discussions with her family members, I decide I want to attempt an intervention. I know I have a small window of time between surgery and treatment. I will need an overnight trip. The only positive here is that it takes me away from thinking about my cancer.

October 12 — My Get the Cancer Out of My Body Day!!
I arrive three hours prior to surgery. Immediately, I am directed to nuclear medicine. The technician injects dye into both breasts. It is a radioactive tracer that moves to the lymph nodes and helps the surgeon identify the sentinel nodes for biopsies. I do not feel any discomfort.

Then I walk to radiology where wires will be placed in both breasts to direct the surgeon to the three tumors. It sounds awful, but it is not. It is an odd experience but done easily and compassionately by the radiologist and her staff. I must wait awhile here before I am wheeled back to surgery.

I entertain myself reading about alcoholism. It is a wonderful distraction.

I now am in the pre-op room. Nurses are prepping me for the surgery. The anesthesiologist arrives. I request no versed. I do not see a reason for taking it. It is the drug that relaxes the patient and causes amnesia. Her facial changes indicate she does not believe it is the right decision for me but will honor it. After more discussion about other topics, she smiles and says, "You don't need versed." I am peaceful about this surgery. I have read about the procedures, discussed them with the surgeon, and believe it will be easy to get through. The surgeon arrives to ask if I have any questions. I share that I do not have appointments with the oncologists. She is surprised and will follow up.

The surgery took two hours for bilateral lumpectomies and sentinel node biopsies. Total time at the hospital was 11 hours. I prepared for a long day and truthfully enjoyed the learning aspect. There was almost no down time. Once ready to go home, the nurse advises me that my urine will be blue from the dye. When dressing, I observe big blue circles on each breast. I love the color and am fascinated. It is a beautiful blue. I have four incisions and many colors on my breasts and underarms. Chunks were taken out of each breast. I am amazed that there are no craters in those areas. Of course, I am swollen. Anna shares the report from the surgeon. All went well.

I come home and feel good. I tell Frank that I did well. He is a bit uneasy. He wants to avoid any conversation. I leave

Wear a bra at night after a lumpectomy. It reduces or eliminates pain.

him with Dee. I go upstairs and make a couple of calls. I try to read but am not focused well. I am too preoccupied. I am reflecting on my day and all that happened to get to this point. When I urinate, I see this gorgeous blue water in the commode. It has me smiling.

In my readings, I learned I should wear a bra to bed after surgery. It will minimize the pain. I only have mild discomfort and go to bed without wearing one. Instantly, I get a high level of pain as I lie on my side. I tolerate it for 30 minutes and realize it will not change. I remember the bra, put it on, lie down, and the pain stops immediately. I sleep reasonably well. It is great information to have. This tip should be in every manual. Yet, I found it in one place on the internet and cannot remember where.

The next day, pain is at a minimum. Tylenol works for me. I have no need for stronger medications. I see the blue in my breasts is less concentrated, and my urine is returning to a normal color. Dang, I was hoping to see it again.

Dee is staying during the day for two more days with Frank. Although I am doing well, I do not want the responsibilities. It is part of my being proactive for a long journey. I stay upstairs and chill out most of the day. Again, I am on the laptop learning more about alcoholism.

October 18
I meet with the radiation oncologist. He has a draft of the pathology results from my surgery and tells me there is no cancer in the lymph nodes. I am celebrating. It indicates there will be no chemotherapy. I can see the end in sight. He sets a two-hour planning meeting for my treatments. However, I need clearance from the medical oncologist before beginning radiation. I do not have that appointment yet.

October 19
I meet with the surgeon for my post-op visit. I am feeling good. The final pathology report states I have early-stage invasive ductal and invasive lobular breast cancers in one breast and invasive lobular cancer in the other one. Micrometastatic

invasive lobular carcinoma, 1 mm in dimension, is found in one sentinel node. These are tiny cancer cells found only because of multiple slices through the node. There is no tumor in the node. I am caught off guard by this finding. It was not in the draft yesterday. It feels like a kick in the stomach. There is more uncertainty again. I am not understanding the implications of it.

I have not been given a date to meet the medical oncologist who works in a different hospital. The office staff has struggled to find the correct number. The surgeon suggests I choose another oncologist and offers some names. I decline. I have made my choice carefully and am not willing to deviate from it.

Every time I think testing is complete, I discover there is another one. The next step is the Oncotype DX test which looks at 17 genes in each tumor. It will tell if I may benefit from chemotherapy and the chances of cancer returning. The results will indicate low, medium, or high risk for recurrence. I am realizing it may be a game changer in my treatment. I hope it is not. The journey has been relatively easy to this point, other than my brain being fatigued from thinking about cancer. It is an adjustment to own cancer. It continues to occupy my mind daily.

The surgeon decides to order the test because of the delay in my getting to the medical oncologist. Normally it is ordered by the oncologist. I am getting highly stressed over the time delay although I understand it will not change anything about my health. Unnecessary time delays frustrate me, knowing I have some cancer cells in my body. I know I have a long journey but truly want it done as soon as possible. The cancer is out, but the remaining treatment will clean up any cancer cells.

After three weeks post-op, my breasts begin itching at the incisions. It is annoying and should not last beyond a few days. Overall, I have found recovery to be easy. Activity is encouraged other than the first two days. My choosing to listen to the surgeon and be receptive to her guidance about activity and arm exercises helped tremendously.

Chemo or Not

Nov. 8

I meet with the medical oncologist. She does not have the results of my test which was ordered by the surgeon last month. She calls and learns the company is waiting for some information. By all available data, she is 95% certain I will not need chemotherapy. There are no indicators at this point. All pathology results work in my favor. She suggests that she call me next week and give me clearance to begin radiation. She is confident and thinks there is no reason for another visit. I am hopeful.

Because of the delays after my surgery, I have some free time. I take a two-night trip to see my friend with alcoholism. It is evident she has cognitive deficits from it. I am heartbroken about her downfall. I become enlightened at the enabling around her. She has no chance of recovery unless the enabling stops. I drive home knowing her decline will continue.

The trip to the OBX also is short. There is minor damage to the beach house from a late October storm. I make a 24-hour trip by myself.

I check on the house and repairs being done, visit friends, and go to one of my favorite restaurants. Of course, I spend a couple of hours on the beach and watch the surfers. It helps me stay balanced and not focus on cancer all day. It also decreases my emotional edge as I wait for these test results.

The same member from church approached me again about joining the breast cancer support group there. I thanked her and explained that my needs are being met, and there is no extra time in my day. Being a full-time caregiver can be consuming. In thinking about this situation, I reflect on how different we all are. We may have a common illness, but our needs are not necessarily the same. What works for some will not work for others. Too often, we forget that part as we attempt to help someone. Perhaps a follow up question is to ask what we can do to support you.

November 24
I have not heard anything from the medical oncologist and was expecting a call last week. It now is Thanksgiving week. I am so frustrated in not being able to get to treatment. I talk with a nurse and learn it is an insurance issue. I call the insurance company. They are not aware of the test being done. The representative calls the surgeon's office and Genomics Health in California. The test has been completed, and results are delayed because of incomplete paperwork by the surgeon's office. They will release the results once they receive the paperwork. The agent with the insurance company tells me she will stay on top of it and keep me informed until I have the results. I am grateful for her support. The test was ordered a few weeks ago and should have been here within 7–10 days. This delay has stressed me. I want to get treatment started and should have by now. I can handle errors in an office, but someone should have called and let me know. The stress is building to a high level. For the first time in this journey, I am on the verge of tears.

I now am understanding better why some patients get frustrated during their health care. It appears that we can be a number and not a person when going through this process. It is not the insurance company. Having cancer is difficult enough. The process should be coordinated and supportive of the patient in the best possible way. There needs to be better customer service in situations like this one.

In recent years, I have learned to be a strong advocate for my health. In some situations, I recognize that I must have someone else take on that responsibility for me. I prefer someone proactive and, when necessary, can be aggressive in advocating. I have friends who get lost in the medical world. I strongly encourage everyone to have a strong advocate with them. Recognize that not all friends can do it. Find the one with this skill set.

Thanksgiving arrives! Frank and I take time to talk about the things that make us smile. I hope to be grateful throughout this journey as the professionals treat my cancer and friends pour their love and support into us. We are blessed in so many ways.

December 2
The insurance representative tells me that results were sent to both the surgeon and medical oncologist two days ago. It is Friday. My surgeon is out of town. The office assistant said, "I can give you a score and nothing else. The score is 24." I know from my reading that 24 means I am an intermediate risk for recurrence. I am thinking the oncologist did not call because she is taking it to the group meeting Monday. The results are not what she expected. These teams of physicians discuss each case and give direction. It is the best thinking of the physicians involved. I like this level of scrutiny and analysis.

I read about the Oncotype DX results online. My score is on the high end in that grouping. There are no long-term studies completed to show if chemotherapy overtreats or no chemotherapy undertreats for someone with an intermediate risk. With the oddities of my cancers, it may not matter.

I begin reading about chemotherapy for early breast cancer. I have put it off until now in hopes it will not be needed. I jot down some questions for the medical oncologist. I decide that if I have a choice, I will go through chemotherapy. I want to maximize my chances of being healthy and being here to care for Frank throughout his life.

December 4
I find it draining to repeat conversations about my health to friends. It also is difficult for me to remember if I have followed through and kept up with everyone. I am too preoccupied. I decide to send group emails. It will help me in multiple ways. When I write down my thoughts, I no longer carry them in my mind. I can clear out the clutter. Additionally, since my free time is limited because of the caregiving, I do not want to be on the phone or laptop constantly. It also limits what Frank may hear about my health.

Here is my first group email:

Cancer Journey Update — December 4

Dear Friends,

I hope you all are enjoying a good day. We attended church this morning, had lunch, and I took a long walk. I needed it.

Several of you have asked for updates. I was hoping I would have more to offer at this point. I discovered the delay was not the insurance company. I called the insurance company, the surgeon's office, and Genomics Health in CA. Once I contacted the insurance company, the rep took a lead role in getting these test results delivered. She knew nothing about it until my call. She was wonderful in keeping me informed of each call she made. My surgeon had not completed the paperwork which held me up for three additional weeks.

The test had been completed but could not be released until all paperwork was filed. The test results were sent via fax and access online to my medical oncologist and surgeon Thursday morning. I have sent emails, called, and received no response. The surgeon is on vacation through the 12th. I have hit my boiling point this weekend. It has been five weeks with a test that at maximum should take ten days.

I have not overly stressed with cancer, the surgery, or any procedures. It is the inexcusable wait times that make this journey difficult. I had surgery eight weeks ago and do not have a plan for further treatment. Treatment should have begun four weeks after surgery. I could go on and on, but I imagine all of you have experienced it at some point in healthcare.

I was able to get a score without other information from the medical assistant to the surgeon at 5 pm Friday. She knew my frustration level. My score puts me in the inter-mediate risk category for cancer appearing elsewhere in my body within ten years. This result was not anticipated by the oncologist. This situation is the one that has no long-term studies to show if chemo overtreats or if no chemo undertreats. I have wrapped my head around the possibility of chemo for the first time. I am hopeful that I will be guided by my best option. If I am put in a position to choose, I will do chemo because of my health and my commitment to Frank.

I am hopeful that I will get clearance to move forward with radiation or have a meeting with the medical oncolo-gist to discuss chemo and begin the process immediately. I am beginning my fifth month with cancer and want to get the treatment started, especially since I have some cancer cells remaining in my body.

Otherwise, all is well with us.

Frank visited Santa. I have attended some UVA basketball games. We are looking forward to friends from Washing-ton state joining us for part of Christmas.

Love,
Marilyn

December 5

The medical oncologist calls and reports that I have an intermediate risk for recurrence. She did not expect this result. She recommends four rounds of chemotherapy, especially with the oddities of my cancer. I have three tumors, two different cancers, and both breasts involved with micro cancer cells in one lymph node. She explains that chemo is a global treatment which kills any remaining cancer cells. She shares information on the drugs and procedures. I ask what to expect after the infusion. She gives me information about what and when to see side effects in the first 21-day cycle. I ask about attending events with crowds such as church and UVA basketball games. I am surprised that I can go. My immunity system will not be compromised significantly. Wow, those comments are a boost to my mental health. I also ask what I can do to help my recovery. She encourages walking as much as possible to help with fatigue. She asks when I want to start. My response is "today." She gets me scheduled for my first infusion four days later. She orders two medications for nausea, so I can get them prior to my big day.

After hanging up the phone, I sit in silence and attempt to grasp the magnitude of changes coming. It is a huge game changer. Now I need a plan for getting Frank and me through this next part of my cancer journey. It will be challenging for both of us. I only wish I could protect him more from what is coming. I know both of us will need support during this treatment process.

I call a couple of friends to process this information. I then call June and Candy about their chemo experiences and discuss it in more depth. I am grateful to have them walking this journey with me. Their personal stories help me navigate this upcoming treatment. I like hearing two different experiences. Best of all, I know I can call them at any time. They have been there. They know what I am facing.

In thinking about the delay with my test results, I honestly believe it is because I chose to work with two different hospitals. If I had stayed with one hospital, I doubt the delay would have occurred. The surgeon only ordered the test because of the delay in getting an appointment with the oncologist. Normally, the oncologist orders that test. The surgeon and staff have been efficient in every other way. However, I know I made the right decision for me by using both facilities.

Chemo Coming Friday — December 7

Dear Friends,

I have a start date for my first chemo treatment. I will meet with the medical oncologist Friday morning (9th) and have a "wonderful" three hours there. Anna will be with me. I think I am ready for it but will learn as I go. I am hoping this journey will be uneventful other than eventually losing my hair. I am not sure how I will respond to that reality.

I did share more information with Frank today. He bowed his head, put his hands on top of his head, and said to take it out. It was his typical reaction to a health situation. He has experienced it too often. A couple of friends at church tonight reinforced that Sis will be okay. Sometimes I am not sure if my stress is my situation or the worry with him. I do know we will get through it well. We always do!

Thank you for your prayers and continuing support. Onward with the treatment plan!

Love,
Marilyn

Comments from friends keep me going. I am including a few of the posts.

"My heart from Winnie the Pooh: You are braver than you believe, stronger than you seem, and smarter than you think. You guys totally have this!"

"You were in my heart as I went to sleep last night.... I will pray for you to be able to support Frank during this time. Your friends will rally around you with so much love and support. You will feel this power throughout the coming weeks. Sending hope and many hugs."

"Great news. Let's get started! You will be through before you know it. Frank will rise to the occasion, I know. Prayers will be with you both!"

"Just a little reminder that I am praying for you and will be praying particularly for tomorrow as you begin your treatments...and your journey to being well again. I will also be praying for Frank. Let us know how it goes."

I get a plan with Dee where she will be with Frank more days. I am attempting to have time without caregiving responsibilities and time for Frank to get out of the house and do other activities. I know these upcoming weeks are going to be extremely difficult for Frank. I will lose my hair which will jolt him.

I am enjoying these few days before chemo. I continue doing what is important to me and remain thankful for the tumors being identified and the care I have received. I have no clue how I will respond to chemo. I have no time to be overwhelmed. I intend to show up and go forward.

Friends encourage, support, and are present in so many ways. Every gesture, no matter how small, impacts me deeply. I am grateful for these friendships. Anna has offered to be with me during my infusions. Her presence provides me with a safety net.

Chemo day has arrived! I have an eye appointment in the morning and am due to be at the infusion center at 1 pm.

I am called for blood work. It will take two hours for the results to be completed. Then the calculations for my medicines begin. Next, I meet with the nurse practitioner. She reviews my medical history and gives me an opportunity to ask questions. She is helpful and makes herself available throughout the day. The oncologist is onsite.

The chemo rooms are private and placed around the nursing station. The nurses can monitor patients easily. I have a glass door and a curtain to pull across the door if I want that level of privacy. There is ample room for Anna and me. What I enjoy is having a large window with lots of sunlight. I am relaxed, sitting in a reclining chair, and ready to get started.

Every possible precaution is taken to be sure I can handle the chemo. I will receive two chemo drugs during this process. A needle is inserted into my hand with no discomfort. There are two nurses who constantly check and recheck numbers in collaboration with the oncologist prior to my receiving the infusion. It is evident that receiving chemo is serious! Obviously, there is a significant amount of wait time. I am given steroids to counteract possible reactions. The nurses explain what can happen and will monitor closely the initial few minutes. I ask what happens if I do react. In short, all staff will descend on the room and take appropriate measures.

Saline is pushed through the lines. The nurses are preparing the first chemo drug. I turn to Anna and say, "Let the poison begin" as the chemo drip starts. After an hour and completion of the medication, the lines are flushed again. The second drug begins and will be completed in less than an hour. I feel nothing different during the infusion. It is strange. I doubt I have a clue about the significance of these coming side effects.

During the infusion, I can push my IV pole and walk the halls when I need the bathroom or a change of scenery. I get restless with so much sitting. It is a LONG day. Because of the toxicity of the medications, there are extra precautions to take in the bathrooms. Well placed signs are helpful. Snacks are available on a cart in the hallway. Knitted hats placed in a box are free to take. Reality is here. It is a quiet day. Sometimes I attempt to read a short article or chat with Anna. I have no interest in doing anything. Mostly, I look through the windows and try to grasp how my days are going to change. I do not think it is possible at this point. I am unable to concentrate on anything.

Before I depart, a Neulasta patch is placed on my upper arm. At a specified time, I will feel an injection to help stimulate the white blood cells. It is used to decrease the risk of infection.

When the oncologist told me 3 hours for the infusion, it obviously did not include everything else that happens on this day. I know now it will be a full day for the next one.

Today has been easy on my body. I feel good as I leave the infusion center. Once home, I sit with Frank. Now I await the side effects coming! I will be leaving my normal and entering the unknown with this "poison" in my body!

Chemo Update — December 9

Well, it was a long 7 hours. Next time it will be 5 hours if I come the day before for the blood work.

It was an easy day with good care. Anna, who accompanied me, was amazed at my calmness. I can't worry about things I do not control. I think my sense of humor will serve me well. As the drip began, I told Anna the poison was starting. I will have a new normal each day.

I got a hat to wear. Once home, Frank told me I could keep it for a short time. He wants me to get a blue one. I thought the yellow, light green, and white one was good. It was the only one that fit. I know I will have more options. He made it clear that I must wear a hat always. He obviously is not liking this journey.

Frank and I both have been challenged with our health since my retirement. We always come through and will do so this time. I am keeping my calendar clear and taking it one day at a time. I have appreciated your many comments of support. I try to respond but obviously will not get to everyone.

This weekend, I plan to help with an event at church Saturday and Sunday. I plan to keep going on with life until I get a signal to slow down or stop. Happy days ahead!! Next chemo in 3 weeks.

Have a great weekend!

Love,
Marilyn

December 10
Wow, chemo is a SHOCK to my body! I awaken with my stomach rumbling but not recognizing it as nausea or anything I know. I know some nasty stuff is in there. It is bizarre. My feet feel like they are wrapped in bubble wrap. They are not numb but quite weird. I lie in bed for a while to absorb my new reality. Dee is downstairs with Frank.

I continue drinking lots of water as advised. I am due to be at church this afternoon to help a friend catering to 300 tomorrow. I know I need to get up and move. It will be interesting to see how I get through it. After slowly getting showered and dressed, I sit for breakfast. I do not have much of an appetite but know I must eat something. I am in a cautious mode. I am not sure what else I might experience.

I drive to church. I have my water and medications with me and am close to the bathroom. I think I will be okay. I cook many pounds of ground beef, help with clean up, and come home three hours later.

I can't quite absorb the magnitude of this change. The oncologist said to expect nausea for 2-3 days. Fortunately, I am well supplied with medications for it. The overall feeling is strange. I do not know how to describe it. Perhaps, it is my "deer in headlights" reaction. I truly begin looking at hour to hour, no longer day to day, month to month, or longer.

I sleep okay. I am on overload as I constantly think about what is happening within my body. Every waking moment is my trying to adjust. I am probably more cautious than I need to be. I drive to church to assist with lunch preparation for 300 people. Even though I am doing my best to be helpful, my mind is in a different place.

During this first week after the infusion, I planned to walk around the block. I only made it five houses away. It seemed like a wind was blocking me, but there was no wind. I was worn out. Within an hour, the chemo fatigue left my body. It reinforced the message that I should walk as much as possible. It can decrease my fatigue.

This journey has taken a significant change in my daily living.

Post Chemo Update — December 15

Dear Friends,

I apologize for group emails, but it is the easiest way for me to get information to you.

My first chemo was last Friday. I awakened Saturday fully aware of something odd going on in my body. Nausea is the primary side effect. Thankfully, I have medications to lessen it but not eradicate it. Sunday night I woke up to horrible bone pain in my knees and lower legs. It continued for 36 long hours. It was a side effect of the bone marrow injection to stimulate the growth of white blood cells. I hope it is working. It will be a topic of discussion next time, so I come home with medications to prevent or reduce the pain.

Late Tuesday afternoon I felt great. Frank and I shopped and enjoyed dinner out. It was the first time I liked any food. Mistakenly, I thought the next few days might be good. Wednesday afternoon nausea hit again and has not stopped. I can manage it but would prefer not to have this feeling.

Other than one day, I have continued with my activities but at a slower pace. I am walking and getting out each day. Today we went to Suffolk to take Tommie a "drunk" fruitcake. This fruitcake was my Mom's tradition with him. Tommie began working for my family when Frank was born. He is 97 and living independently. We love him dearly and are blessed to spend time with him.

Frank is holding on. He told me one night that he could cry. The upcoming hair loss is scaring him. I am glad he is sharing his feelings and participating in helping me. It is a different chapter for us, but all is well thus far. I try to keep him in his activities and distracted from my health.

Chemo is a roller coaster ride. My chemo targets primarily the hair, stomach, and bowels. I cannot predict day to day or hour to hour. I go with whatever happens. If I need to chill, I do. It is more challenging than I anticipated. I hope this first cycle is the worst other than the cumulative fatigue that will occur. My second session is scheduled for December 28th.

Thank you again for your visits, calls, emails, texts, and cards. Your support keeps me going!

We are hoping to have an extra special Christmas with a visit from our dear friends in Washington state. If they can get a military flight out, we will have them with us. Frank is hyped! I wish you joy and peace throughout the holidays and new year.

Love,
Marilyn

Abbreviated comments:

"Oh, gosh...It sounds like you must feel you have entered a combat zone. Can I bring you something?"

"Your positive attitude is inspirational! You do more for your friends than you know. Sending love and positive thoughts back at you for a Merry Christmas."

"What a trip you are having. I am glad Frank is talking to you about how he feels. I think that helps both of you."

"We hate to think of all the negative effects of the chemo. I guess that's a sign that it is doing something very powerful in a positive way, too."

My good days are not close to normal. Everything in my body has been turned upside down. The changes within my body can drain me at times. It is important that I retain a positive outlook and continue to focus on getting healthy again. It only indicates that I get through my days easier.

Over the weekend I am surprised by three different friends bringing meals. It helps tremendously. I do not have to plan, shop, prepare, or cook. There is so much food that I can freeze some in several small containers. I honestly do not know if I can handle doing it anyway. With Dee helping us more and more, I do not have the pressure of doing it all on my own.

Feeling Good! — December 19

Just a quick note that the bad is over for this cycle! I have enjoyed three good days with no symptoms other than the numbness in my feet. Today I walked two miles at the mall with Caryn. I was surprised the hallways were not crowded.

If the next cycle repeats this one, I will be prepared better for that challenging first week.

I hope you are enjoying the Christmas season.

Love,
Marilyn

Some comments:

Great news!! You really do rock!!

"Praise God! So glad you are feeling good and able to get out with your friend."

"I'm SOOOOOOOOOOOOOOOOOO glad to read this one! Now at least you are prepared for the next battle. Good for you!"

Feeling good means that I can function better for that day. In no way does my body feel anything like it did prior to chemo. There is no description for it. Nothing is normal!

December 24

I love the Christmas season. However, I know I am going through the motions and doing the best I can. It is not our normal. When I am not fully functioning, it always impacts Frank. I see a slip in his thinking and focus. Yet, he remembers to prepare for Santa's arrival by clearing a path to the fireplace and preparing a plate of cookies, a cup of eggnog, and a bunch of carrots. He tells me what to write on a note for Santa. Thankfully, I took care of the shopping and wrapping early this year.

December 25

I awaken and see lots of hair on my pillowcase. It is not going to be an enjoyable part of this journey. Merry Christmas! I am wondering how quickly I will lose my hair. Will it come out in ugly clumps? Will it evolve slowly? Will I change my mind and get it shaved? I get a vacuum cleaner and keep it in my bedroom. My intent is to vacuum my bedroom and bathroom and put a hat on for the rest of the day. Reality is here. The side effects of chemo can be difficult. Living through each day takes everything I have.

The days before and after Christmas are quiet. I do not have extra energy. I feel like I am going through the motions and not truly enjoying this season. Chemo is controlling my body.

I have walked forty-five minutes most days. I am not moving at my fast pace, maybe more out of a caution with my feet. I have been able to keep up with the few activities on my calendar and continue to limit what I will schedule. My calendar is bare compared to life before chemo.

Advice during chemo:

Walk, walk, walk —
It reduces fatigue.

47

Chemo #2 — December 27

Hi to All,

I hope everyone had a wonderful Christmas! I had a great second week after my treatment and was able to enjoy Christmas with Frank and friends. Annoying symptoms returned but did not keep me down. On Christmas day my hair began to shed strands. I must wear a hat to keep my hair from falling into the food. It reminds of my time with our German Shepherd. I would clean the house, and, within hours, her shedding was noticeable. Now it is my turn. In talking with others, I am learning that this shedding drove them crazy. It is what led them to get their heads shaved. When I asked how they felt when getting it shaved, they all said they were traumatized. My hair stylist validated that reaction and discouraged my going that route. I have no need to be traumatized. I plan to wear a hat and empty it out each day until there is no more. I have never liked wearing hats but will learn to love them in this situation.

This third week is not as easy as the second week. The scalp pain increases day by day as it prepares to let my hair go. I have not brushed my hair for many days. Nausea and a metallic taste have returned and are eased by medications. The bottoms of my feet are weird and have been since the first day. It feels like I am walking on air mattresses. Sometimes it gets painful. It changes my gait. I now wear shoes for stability all day. Normally, I am without shoes in my home. I have endured over 30 surgeries, mostly orthopedic, and none of it compares to this experience. I truly have a poison in my body. It reminds me daily of its presence, even on good days. I have a great ability to block out and move on. These symptoms are too powerful to block out. I am learning to live with them, use medications more aggressively to combat the symptoms, and keep on living life as I want in a modified way. My new normal continues to change day to day.

Once I have no hair, I will be fitted for a wig. I may try something quite different. Seize the opportunity! I also have learned there is a strong probability that my auburn hair may not return as the same color or texture. It will be interesting!

Frank is holding up well. If he hears me talking about my health, he goes elsewhere to avoid it. The big test will be my upcoming baldness. I think these last weeks have helped prepare me. I may be blown away when it happens. Who knows! I have been blessed by not having anger, denial, or grief so far. I am more concerned about understanding what is happening at every step. I don't know how people get through these journeys without being grounded in their faith and having supportive family and friends. I have no fear with my health. I just want to get the best possible care for a long-term health outcome.

Tomorrow I will have my second chemo treatment. I expect this day to go smoothly. It will be the next day that my body will be exploding with awful symptoms. Sitting at home is not good for me unless the symptoms demand it. Last time I only had two days I was shut down. I have some fatigue in my legs and expect it to get worse in the weeks to come. I have kept a journal and will see if the pattern repeats.

I have events planned for the weekend but imagine it will be hour by hour decisions to go or not. I wish each of you a Happy, Healthy New Year. I plan to have a great year despite this breast cancer journey! Each day is a day closer to being free of cancer.

By the way, I have appreciated the prayers, communications, visits, and meals. They get me through my days. Thank you! I am blessed to have a wonderful group of friends to walk this journey with me. It is a journey that cannot be done alone. So, onward I go.

Love,
Marilyn

Replies from friends keep me going. Here are two:

"Hopefully you are waking up to a better day. Thank you for documenting your journey. It gives me a lot of insight for my rare patients who are undergoing chemo but also empathy in general towards others.

You'll continue to be in my daily prayers and thoughts as will Frank. He's found a coping mechanism that works for him (general avoidance when it gets to be too much) which I love in so many ways because of its evolutionary origin and its proven track record. (It's HOT – don't touch it, it's TOO BRIGHT – don't look at it, that HURTS – don't do it again!!). And it is what children do to cope in so many ways. I love that you are letting him talk when he needs to and letting him walk away when he needs to. You're both doing well. Hopefully, this is your incredibly strong body reacting just as it should to this life-saving poison.

Keep your ever-present, "Marilyn-defining," God-given-gift-of-extreme-perseverance. I don't ever believe that God does things like cancer to people, but I do believe that our lives prepare us for certain experiences. In some ways, you have been very, very well prepared for this. Doesn't make it much easier though."

"Love to you, my friend! If attitude is the key to becoming cancer free, you'll be a winner for sure. You are an inspiration! Peace and prayers! Hugs! "

I decide to get my bloodwork done a day before my second infusion. I walk in, sign my name, get called immediately, and go home within minutes. It will save me two hours on the infusion day. It is well worth the trip here. Tonight, I can see the results in my patient portal. I like this instant access to my medical information.

I meet with the oncologist during each infusion. I inquire about options for preventing or coping with the bone pain from the patch. She gives me options such as Claritin or an anti-inflammatory to prevent the pain. I am taking Claritin daily with no impact. I will be ready to attack it this time by using a different medication. Once again, I am appreciative of the support I receive during these visits. The oncologist reinforces what I am doing well and offers suggestions to help me with concerns. She always gives me the time I need.

Chemo #2 Update — January 3

Hi Everyone,

I had my second infusion last Wednesday. I came home and walked 50 minutes. It felt great. Reality hit me the next day. I was armed with medicines and stayed on top of the symptoms. Like clockwork, my body loudly announced it was time for medicine to prevent nausea. It is unlike anything I have experienced. I had a bad taste in my mouth 24/7. Distractions helped. Sucking on hard peppermint candy helped. My feet are partially numb. The good news is I no longer feel like I am walking on air mattresses. My balance is better. My fingers have lost sensation. The skin on my fingers is cracking despite cream recommended for it.

On Saturday I drove to Charlottesville for the UVA game. My medicine for bone pain worked. I was confident I could make it. On the drive home, I struggled to stay awake during the last 30 minutes. I did not expect the fatigue to return. I neglected to think about that part. I came home, slept for two hours, and went next door for a party. The fatigue was huge on Sunday. I made it to church and later took a few decorations upstairs. Climbing the stairs was challenging. I knew I needed to walk and kept putting it off. It took me 28 minutes to walk a course in the neighborhood that normally takes 15 minutes. Only by talking to a friend on the phone during my walk was I able to complete the walk.

On Monday two friends from church came to visit. Carolyn crocheted a beautiful prayer shawl for me. Joanne made a beautiful prayer cross which can be used as a bookmark for Frank. It was special! Additionally, Carolyn left us a container of homemade chicken soup which is delicious. As Frank says when he likes something, it is "good stuff". I truly enjoyed my visit with them.

I have been offered help with the Christmas decorations, but keep remembering my oncologist saying to push through the fatigue and stay active. Getting the decorations upstairs and packed gives me a purpose while I am in the house. I work for a few minutes and take a break. The best part is I know every day is a day closer to good health, and treatment is done! By night time, the fatigue has lifted. I can climb the stairs and not think about it. It is weird how the fatigue comes and goes so strongly and quickly. The big black cloud envelopes me, stays for a couple of days, and rapidly leaves.

I have some hair on my head. Every day I deal with clumps coming out and having to vacuum it up. I jammed the vacuum cleaner once. I try to confine it to my bedroom and bathroom. My thick hair is now quite thin. I wear a hat to keep from dealing with hair flying everywhere. I am ready to get through this stage. The scalp pain has calmed down.

Today I have a physical therapy appointment. It is not related to my cancer treatment. I continue to plan one day at a time. Soon I should be dealing with 24-48 hours of fatigue again. When these strong symptoms become quieter, then I can look forward to going out more and meeting friends.

I am hopeful I will have two reasonably good weeks prior to my third treatment. I remain grateful to the physicians and support staff who diagnosed my cancers, performed procedures and surgeries to identify the cancers and remove the tumors, and provided treatment to kill whatever cancer may be elsewhere in my body. I remain optimistic and continue to be thankful for my friends who have supported both Frank and me. I am grateful for each day.

For those of you not on my Facebook page, at church Sunday, Frank decided he needed to help the Pastor with communion. He got up from his seat and stood by Pastor Mark. When I went up for communion, I looked at Frank. With a smile on his face, he motioned that he and Mark were tight. I don't think Mark had seen this side of Frank. At the end of the service, I watched him get up again when he heard the beginning of "Go Tell It on The Mountain" played and sang by three musicians. Frank stood in front, pretended to hold a "mike", sang the song, and directed the congregation. I was in the back of the church and felt my phone vibrate. I had a text. It was a friend near Frank who wanted to be sure I did not miss it. She knew I was preoccupied. Frank is Frank. He lives in the moment. How blessed we are to be with a church where he can worship in his unique ways. Even more special this time, I was sitting with the Judge who approved my guardianship and granted Frank the right to vote in 2003. Only in the past year did I realize he was our Judge. He talked about Frank and cheered him on throughout this service. He said watching Frank each Sunday is a highlight for him. Frank is teaching all of us! When I asked Frank why he did it, he said Andy (Griffith) and God were in his ear and told him to do it. At least, he included God. I am honored to be his sister and so proud of his confidence and belief in self.

After church, a friend was teasing me about my hat and loss of hair. Frank intervened and told him over and over " kind, kind, kind". Then Frank told him to give me a hug. Wow, what a protective brother! Of course, at home, he called me Ms. Kojak which made me burst out laughing. Frank can tease me, but don't let someone else do it during this journey.

I hope you are having a great start to this new year! I am thriving with your support!

Love,
Marilyn

More comments:

"Keep up the good fight. See u both Friday".

"Marilyn, the emails describing your journey through chemo and life, as it is, have really captured my attention. — Your faith, hope, and the love you have from so many must be a boost to your spirits and recovery."

"I love this friendship update. Have you ever written a book? If not, you should."

I do not have a port for my chemo. It was never discussed. It has worked well for me without it. It is one less outpatient procedure and less stress. I am comfortable with the needles. There are only two with each infusion, one for the blood work and one in my hand for the chemo drugs. It will be a total of eight sticks in twelve weeks. Not bad! I have friends who had a port and never knew it was a choice. I am thankful it was not expected. Had my veins collapsed, then I imagine I would have needed a port.

Update on Chemo #2 — January 7

Dear Friends.

I went to church Wednesday. I mostly sat because of my fatigue and helped a bit with clean up. Cold symptoms bothered me all day. The oncologist said days 7-10 are days with my lowest immunity. Thursday was day 8. It is the day in both cycles when I had a breakthrough with my symptoms. They either lower in intensity or disappear. This time, I began to feel the best yet. I went to physical therapy with some fatigue in the morning, came home to have lunch with Frank, walked 40 minutes, and went out to dinner. I had ample energy that evening. It was remarkable when I consider the previous week.

My hair has been falling out for 14 days. I am intrigued by the change. The hair is pitiful looking. I easily can count the few strands remaining. It has eased me into acceptance of being bald. I wear a hat from morning till night and only put it on and take it off in my bedroom. It controls the damage from the shedding. I have grown tired of vacuuming my pillow, floors, and tub daily, but am glad I chose not to have my head shaved. I have not experienced any trauma at this point. I know it is temporary. It is a small price to pay for potentially life-saving procedures. Frank walked by me (hat on) and told me I had a bald spot. Good for him! We both need to laugh. Up until this point, he has been in avoidance mode with my hair.

Yesterday was awesome! I felt great! I did have side effects but did not think about them. PROGRESS! Dee had Frank. I had a day of no responsibility. We were treated to a home-cooked meal. We have another one for the weekend. Our church is providing some meals this month. Other friends are helping, too. It is the first time I have ever been in a position of need to this level. The meals eliminate my having to plan, buy, and prepare. What a gift! It takes that stressor off my plate. It is the overall fatigue that requires me to do less and preserve my energy. If I had to take on "normal" responsibilities, I would struggle and fail. It takes a village to get one through chemo. I have been blessed in so many ways with friends helping us.

I put my snow flag up on January 1. Can I take responsibility for this incoming snow??? I LOVE snow. I went to the mailbox and got the paper this morning. That short walk was an eye-opener. My body is not close to what it was before I started chemo. I got winded. Of course, my cold is a contributor. I was hoping to drive to the reservoir and take pictures later today but may have to hold back on that thought.

I must say Frank has risen to his highest level of helping without my asking. I love the way he has helped and protected his Sis. He has been coached well by our close friends. He met with the counselor this week and surprised her with his confidence. Apparently, he talked the entire time. I hear it daily, but the counselor had not experienced him talking that freely. He is beginning to understand that I want him to have someone else with whom he can talk about anything. I love watching the growth in Frank. He is an amazing man! Yes, I am biased!!!!

My thinking at this point is I will have mostly good days before my next infusion. There will be some bumps along the way, but I should be able to handle them. I hope to get a wig. Won't it be interesting to see how this event will turn out?! If the pattern of side effects continues, I only will have one week of difficulty after each of the next two infusions. I can handle it! Of course, the accumulation of fatigue and possibility of chemo brain are the unknowns.

We got the call that our friends from Washington state landed at Andrews AFB yesterday afternoon. There have been no flights from their area to the east coast since mid-December. They will arrive at our home Monday. Frank and I are excited and ready to have them here.

I plan to enjoy my good days until the next infusion on the 18th. A good day means the side effects are not screaming at me. Again, I continue to be grateful and sometimes overwhelmed at the support you are providing me. THANK YOU!

ENJOY THE SNOW!!

Love,
Marilyn

I have taken some selfies to send my friends in Washington. It gives them a reality check of my physical state. My head is skimpy with a few strands of hair standing up. What an adjustment! I think I am getting through it well but without enjoyment. I could never have imagined I would be going through this treatment and having to deal with total hair loss. Before I leave my bedroom, I put a hat on so Frank will not have to see my drastically changed look.

I have been blessed to have friends constantly check in with me. These frequent calls and visits mean so much in getting me through each day. This journey with chemo is difficult. I cannot imagine going through this treatment without this loving support.

Positive Attitude Conquers All! — January 17

Dear Friends,

Sunday, we went to church. Once home I sat non-productively for too long and decided to go walk. With fatigue, it means I must push myself to go out even though I love walking. As I began, I made the decision to do my normal 2.5-mile walk. It was my first attempt at this route in six weeks. It has some hills. I did not know if the fatigue would stop me, but I had to try it. I had my phone to call someone if needed. Happily, I can report that I did it with ease. I was thrilled. Two weeks ago, I could hardly walk around the block without great effort. I like these recovery days when I can do more. I also was less tired that evening. It is true that walking makes one less tired during chemo. It is imperative that I walk as much as possible even though my body may be rebelling.

Someone at church surprised me with two new hats. Eventually, I might be able to color coordinate with my clothes. I am continuing to adjust to having to wear a hat all day. My body temperature seems to be warmer. I do not require the layers of clothes that I normally would use with this weather.

I left a message for the wig lady and am waiting for an appointment. My hair is skimpy. It takes 5 seconds or less to dry it. I look like one of the Three Stooges with his wild hair in all directions. Not attractive, I might say! My eyebrows and eyelashes are still with me. Apparently, they may go after all chemo.

Our friends from Washington state come at a great time. I am down with a horrible cold. Dean works on my honey-do list, including installing a new microwave. Mary Louise takes over meal preparation, care for Frank, and anything else that needs to be done. We have a wonderful visit. Mary Louise and I are childhood friends.

I received a call recently from someone who said, "I heard you were sick." My immediate response was "No, I am not sick." I have never considered myself to be sick because of treatment. It has not crossed my mind. I certainly have limitations. It took me by surprise. I think I like my perspective better. It is a mind game getting through this treatment.

Overall, this second cycle has been easier. I knew what to expect and did a better job handling some of the side effects. The big change has been an increase in daily fatigue. At times it has shut me down, mostly in the week after infusion. I schedule only one event per day with rare exception. It gives me time to be with Frank, chill, and get a 30-minute walk done on most days. From my old normal, it is a SLOW day. With this new normal, it does not seem slow. It just takes longer to do what I want. Often my short to-do list does not get done. It does not seem to matter. There is always another day to do it. I think I have adapted well to conserve my energy. Extra sleep does not help. I awaken tired and go to sleep exhausted many nights. Naps have no impact on chemo fatigue. This, too, shall pass.

Frank and I went to a 4 pm movie one day. I struggled to stay awake. It was another example of a surprise attack with chemo fatigue. I never know when it might hit me.

Despite the fatigue, my spirits are good. I have not had a mentally down day. I know this stuff is temporary. I work with what I have and enjoy my day. I just want to do everything possible to kick this cancer!

I began taking steroids today in preparation for the "poison" tomorrow. I had my lab work done this morning. I am having to psych myself up to endure the following seven days. Chemo is a jolt to my system and not enjoyable. Thank goodness there are two decent weeks after the bad week before the next cycle. So, two cycles down and two to go! I can see the light at the end of the chemo tunnel!!

Thanks again for all you are doing to support Frank and me!

Love,
Marilyn

Some comments to my email:

"I type this on a plane knowing that today is your chemo day. I hope it went well. I must say, YOUR positive attitude conquers again! It is heart-warming to hear that your walks are getting better with time. Of course, I realize by the time you receive this, you may not feel like taking another walk – but you know you will be able to in a matter of days. And you are a short-timer as we said when I served in the US Army whenever a fellow soldier was getting close to concluding his service. Your "service" in therapy is half-way over. Great marker! I can't wait to see some of your hats. My thoughts and prayers are with you, my friend!!"

"LOVE hearing your positivity. It TRULY is inspirational. We hope you know how meaningful your life is to others. Can't wait to see you tomorrow. I'll be there with bells on!!!!"

"I am so proud of you! Your attitude is so positive. You go girl!!!

"Marilyn, I love reading this but more than anything enjoyed your company today. You glowed today – which isn't really expected with all you're going through. Your positive energy radiates."

"You are such an inspiration to us all on the island. I will read Dad your email for he asks about you and Frank often. I pray this third round will be a bit less invasive and doesn't bring your energy down as much. It is wonderful that you are able to continue your daily walks on most days."

I finally realized that I was fighting a bacterial infection and not a cold. It took three prescriptions to manage it. During that period, it snowed. For the first time ever, I did not have the energy to get off the sofa and walk to the window to see it. Normally, I am outside taking pictures and embracing it. That infection on top of the chemo caused some tough days for me.

Three Down and One to Go! — January 23

Dear Friends,

I had an annual visit with a physician. I was wearing a hat. He said, "Is it so cold you need to wear a hat inside now?" I removed my hat and surprised him. He had no clue. His comment was, "You look too good to be going through chemo." I have heard this statement several times. I hope it is true. I do not want to "wear" my chemo.

How do I say I enjoyed my chemo day last week?! A friend who taught with me at an elementary school in the mid-80s spent the day with me. As we walked in, someone heard my name, looked at me and told me I taught her son (in the 80's). I looked at Debbie as we walked down the hall and said, "That is Kit, a parent of students at our school." After I got settled, I took my IV pole and went looking for her. She was helping another parent we knew in an adjacent room. We spent time catching up with their families and neighbors. The day became all social. Debbie and I had lots of catching up to do as well. There was no downtime and no thinking about chemo. It was a blast from the past. I might note that I do not have any side effects when receiving chemo. It has been an easy day each time other than knowing poison is being dumped into my body. Friends accompanying me keep me from thinking too much about it.

In my chat with the oncologist, she said I was one of her models for dealing with chemo. She does not think my fatigue will increase because of the way I am handling it. I hope she is right. Isn't it amazing that I can control the severity of the cumulative fatigue with my walking?! I shared that last time the bad fatigue hit on my return from UVA, and I wanted to know how I could avoid it. I was not safe driving the last thirty minutes. Obviously, I want to go to the game in three days this time. She said the fatigue crash was due to my coming off steroids and not from the Neulasta patch. Since I was not having any issues, she told me to stop the steroids. Now my fatigue should hit Friday which will free me for the Saturday game. I like her thinking!!

I have revised my approach to this cycle. On my good days, I plan to push and see what I can do. It will not look like my old normal since I am rarely preparing meals and no longer traveling. I did a test the day before chemo. I pushed myself all day and felt good. The reward that evening was no fatigue. I was not tired at bedtime. It once again reinforces the necessity of being active to eliminate some of the fatigue. It works every time. It is amazing to experience it. If I sit and do nothing, the fatigue can shut me down. It becomes a mind game, and I plan to win on most days. It is a fight. If I did not love physical activity, this journey would be much more difficult.

Based on my two previous cycles, I should be experiencing strong symptoms. Surprise....the symptoms are not the same. The nausea is playing out differently this time. I am getting headaches and feel like I will throw up. Medicines help but do not eliminate the feeling. This part of the chemo is the hardest. I can function but not focus well. Frank and I ran a few errands. Then I was done. Thankfully, our fridge is full of food. All I must do is heat up something.

Two days away and the fatigue crash hit hard, just like the oncologist anticipated. For the first time, I went to bed during the day. I was out of it for a couple of hours.

The next day I made it to the UVA game. The fatigue had lifted. However, my feet and lower legs were numb. I had to watch where I was walking to be sure I maintained my balance. I took my time. Walking the incline to the arena felt like climbing a mountain. I was winded. I also had that yucky taste. It was not metallic, but bad. I kept peppermints in my pocket and sucked on them. I enjoyed the game despite these side effects, and UVA won. I treated myself to a peppermint milkshake for the trip home and still lost a pound that day. I did not want one second with that horrible chemo taste.

My body temperature continues to be higher. I now sleep with no covers which is totally unlike me. I awaken most nights because I am hot. I guess they are hot flashes which I did not have prior to chemo. It is weird. I love burning wood in the fireplace. Because of my temperature change, there have been no fires since mid-December.

Four days out and I awakened with less numbness in my lower legs. Now the forefoot of each foot is numb. We made it to church and got a walk done later. I had to push myself to complete 30 minutes. I made it. The bad taste is less offensive. It is a good thing there are good days before another round of chemo. It gives me a chance to forget the bad and enjoy the good. These first few days are not to be cherished. Thankfully, I only have one more week of this stuff after I get through the next few days. I would not wish it on anyone.

I decided to order a wig I have been seeing for several weeks. It is made by a company used by the American Cancer Society. I went online and learned there was a huge warehouse fire. No wigs are available currently. Oh well! I am tired of the hats and probably will have the same feeling about the wig. I find I need some hatless time and must ask Frank not to come in the living room for a period. It gives my head the break it needs. Yes, I do have some hair. The oncologist does not expect me to lose anymore. It is pitiful but better than none. My standards have changed out of necessity.

Yesterday we were treated to another wonderful home-cooked dinner. These meals have made a huge difference in my getting through each day. I cannot imagine having to assume all responsibilities during chemo treatment. Thank you to everyone involved!

Today we are greeted with more rain. Now I must figure out where I can walk. It is not an option. I continue with the numbness in my feet and a milder chemo taste. I have not taken nausea medicine for 24 hours. It is a good sign, but I realize nausea can return. Getting out and doing something keeps me from focusing on these side effects. Hopefully, I will have only one more day of these bad side effects.

The day prior to my infusion, I had lunch with my radiologist. She is a rare physician who truly listens to her patients and works to make significant changes to improve patient care and not only in her department. She has been the guiding light in my breast cancer journey. I have the highest respect for her work and have been fortunate to have her as one of my physicians! As I shared with her, my view of a radiologist's role has changed dramatically. How can I complain about my journey when I have exceptional physicians working with me?! They are a huge part of my optimism and determination to live each day and not let breast cancer define me.

Despite the ugliness of breast cancer, I feel blessed in multiple ways. I think I have found a way to make lemonade out of the lousy lemons. My journey is a success because of the widespread support I have received from friends and professionals. I thank you daily for your part in my life and the support you give both Frank and me. I treasure it.

I hope you are having a great start to the week.

Love,
Marilyn

The family sitting next to me at the UVA games has invited me to ride with them to Charlottesville on game days. It is a fun group, and it allows me to enjoy the game days more. The long drives take so much effort to concentrate on what I am doing. Now I can cast worries aside and be in the moment. The timing of this invitation is wonderful. I do not think they know how much I am challenged on these days. I watch the game but certainly do not take in what I would without the effects of chemo.

Have a New Look — January 29

Dear Friends,

Well, I visited the wig salon at the hospital. I was surprised. There is a room dedicated to it. There is a chair like ones I sit in for my hair cuts. Mirrors surround the chair. Wigs are on display. It is an inviting environment with a wonderful resource person to assist. She is well suited for this job. Wigs are new and provided via a grant. In contrast, my community hospital is run by volunteers doing their best to help you find a used wig. I also took time to browse the resource center. There was good information available.

I was determined to have fun and try something different. First, she wanted me to try a blond wig. The hair was too perfect looking. I don't think I am cut out to be a blond or have a perfect style. I told her I needed a rumpled look. I spotted a strawberry blond wig with some highlights. I liked it. The color is closer to the bright carrot top from my childhood. We laughed and chatted more. Three hours and time to go home!

The first week after chemo continues to be challenging. I do believe I got through it better by pushing myself more during the day. It decreases the fatigue which is quite noticeable when staying in the house so much. On this round, the bad symptoms subsided a day earlier. Now I am wondering if it is because of my increase in overall activity. On days 7–8, I moved constantly. By 10 pm, I was unable to function any longer. I am feeling great about my journey thus far and am somewhat relieved I am closer to the finish line. Until now, I have not allowed myself to think about the end of treatment. It is in sight which means I can think about returning to the beach.

Hiring a caregiver for Frank has made a huge difference in my getting through each week. It gives me time to back away from my responsibilities. Frank sees it as an uplifting time for him since he will do different things. We are blessed to have Dee in our lives.

In my first good week, I met a friend for lunch and a movie. The following day I attended the Richmond Symphony in Powhatan. Oh, it feels good to be doing normal activities again. It stretches me. I always know the chemo is in my body. Again, I cannot reiterate enough about the mindset. I think the one symptom that continues to affect me daily is the numbness in my feet. When I walk my balance is off. One day I went looking for bald eagles at the reservoir. With camera in hand, I had to think about my walking. I must pay attention. Shopping at the grocery store is easier because I can hold onto the basket. Rarely will I use the small hand baskets now. When taking a long walk, I use a walking pole. The pole negates the balance issue. Often there are solutions to my concerns. It requires me to think outside of the box and not manage things out of habit.

I have been surprised at some of the responses I receive from these emails. My wonderful radiologist and several of you have encouraged me to write a book. I cannot imagine doing it. Who would want to read it? My standard answer has been, "It is not on my bucket list". When I chatted with the resource person who fitted me with a wig, she pushed hard for me to write. She said patients need to hear stories of cancer patients getting through it and dealing with it in a positive way. Since I am more focused on reading the facts and not stories, I have stayed away from it. I have appreciated the compliments and have been overwhelmed with many of your comments.

Hugs and love,
Marilyn

Comments:

"You look great. I love your new look."

"I LOVE IT. You'd look beautiful ANY OL' way because YOU ARE, but I love it."

I have stayed with my plan to focus on one day at a time. So far, it is working. It takes all my energy to get through each day and have some time with Frank. I am blessed to receive so much positive support from my friends. My physicians are encouraging but never lead me to think it is done. This journey is long with chemo. The cumulative fatigue begins to kick in. My thinking is not as sharp. I know I cannot handle a normal day.

Throughout the weeks of dealing with chemo, I think about it all day. My body internally is so strange. Nothing is normal. I cannot get away from it. I am not worried. I am trying to focus on getting well. It takes everything I have to stay positive and focus on the good. The reality of this long journey has given me a deeper understanding. With chemo, it seems to be a good twelve to eighteen months from diagnosis to being recovered. I may need to reevaluate after radiation.

My weight varies within six to seven pounds during each cycle. I lose weight during the week of the infusion. Because of the meals being brought to us, my weight returns to my baseline. If these meals were not available, I would not eat properly. I know they have contributed to my remaining reasonably healthy during my treatment.

No More Chemo!!! — February 9

Dear Friends,

In the past two months, I think I have cooked only two meals. We have been so fortunate to have friends show up with meals. We have eaten well. Not only has it saved my energy, but it has made me more willing to eat with these side effects. The food is there. It is wonderful. I don't have to do anything but sit down and enjoy. What a blessing! For now, I need to clean out the freezer and see what I can handle.

I think this journey has opened my eyes more than ever about the depth of friendships. Frank has been with me for 17 years. In recent years his needs have become more demanding. I have put him first and lacked time to see friends. It has overwhelmed me to see so many friends come forward to help me. It also is the first time in my life that I have been in a position that I would not be able to go forward without help. This journey is unpredictable and not one that I could have planned what I needed. It could have become concerning since there is no other adult in the house to take on a major role. I am deeply grateful to everyone who has supported us in any way. Every gesture has been heartfelt and made a difference in my health. I get a bit teary thinking about all of you and your impact. I have remained positive which is my way. However, I have never had to work on it because of my support system. Please don't ever underestimate what your kind gestures, no matter how small, do for someone in true need. It also has given me more opportunity to talk with Frank about the continuing need to help others and why we do it.

My two recovery weeks with the third cycle were good. I decided to push myself closer to a normal day. For those of you who know me well, you know I must push the limits at some point. I pushed too hard and finally found a middle ground. I continue with neuropathy in my hands and feet, a slight balance and gait issue, a level of fatigue that keeps me from going full force, an inability to eat anything with vinegar because of the damage to my stomach, a rash on my legs and arms, and a feeling of my teeth not being cleaned. By now, I do not focus solely on them. I had days where chemo was not my primary thought. I continue to drive, and I have avoided chemo brain so far.

June brought a meal and flowers which made me think about each day getting closer to treatment ending. Until now I have not looked beyond the present day or week. Spring is coming. I look forward to returning to the beach.

I have received my last infusion and am celebrating. I received a certificate of completion and got to ring the bell as I walked out. It was a wonderful feeling! I had good care at the infusion center. I will return to my local hospital for radiation. Now I am focused on getting my body restored after the four rounds of chemo.

Today has been my best first day after an infusion. My body has adjusted to this "poison." I am taking it easy for a few days and hoping to catch up on paperwork at home. This is my "tough it out" week with the chemo taste. At least I know there is an ending to it.

Thanks again for all you have done to support me during my breast cancer journey. I am closing the chemo chapter and will be ready to move to the next treatment phase soon.

Love,
Marilyn

More comments:

"Hey, Marilyn-
GRRRRRRRRRRRRRRRRRRRRRRRRRRRRRRRRRRRRRREAT to hear this news! You continue to defy the "norm" in your own positive way. Bravo to you, my friend, for maintaining a balance in so many aspects of your life... no matter what is thrown your way. I continue to be VERY proud of you!
Hugs"

'Loved seeing the picture of your ringing the bell and rejoicing. I rejoice, too!! WOO HOO We must celebrate!"

"This is the best news I've heard in a long time. Congrats and I'm humbled by your attitude and bravery with all of this."

"I love to read your updates. It is much better than the notes I receive from your treating physicians. Hearing what actually happens behind the scenes is eye-opening."

Time to Resest and Begin My Recovery — February 18

To My Exceptionally Supportive Friends,

Oh my, this fourth cycle knocked me off my feet for a few days. I guess I blocked it out each cycle and am surprised when it happens again. I had zero energy and could not get going. On day five, I felt somewhat human again. All food tasted extremely salty. Nothing quenched that thirst. I am thrilled I will not have to go through this ugliness again. Chemo is unlike anything I have ever experienced. My insides have been damaged. I know it will take more time to restore my health.

With the 80-degree weather, I was wearing shorts during my walk. With the wind blowing, it felt like feathers constantly brushing against my lower legs. WEIRD! I could not feel the wind. My feet seem worse. As in the first round, it feels like I am walking on an air mattress. My hands have lost some sensation. I struggle turning pages and picking up small items. I hope this neuropathy will resolve soon.

Food does not taste normal. It can be good but not like it was pre-chemo. I graze all day to deal with the chemo taste. Fortunately, I have not gained weight. I have learned what foods work best for me and what to avoid. I put a temporary stop to meals coming in. I have too much food here. We had shrimp one evening. I tasted one and thought my mouth was on fire. The Old Bay did not work well for me. I keep trying. Anything with any level of spice is off my list. Some days I cannot tolerate something. Days later, the same food is agreeable. I have learned to adapt to whatever as it occurs. When I get to the recovery days, the food is better. I long for my pre-chemo taste again. Now that chemo is done, I can look back and see the incredible impact on my body. Yes, it kills cancer. Yes, the body pays a huge price! Yes, I will be healthy again! Yes, it was worth going through!

On a brighter note, my hair began growing again two weeks ago. It is earlier than anticipated. It is a pleasant surprise. At this point, the coloring and texture appear to be the same as before. Only time will tell the true outcome.

I think the biggest challenge has been staying strong mentally, especially when there have been non-functioning hours/days. I am thankful those days are behind me. I have learned so much and have a deeper understanding and appreciation for anyone going through this journey. It is not easy. I am convinced my knowledge and positive attitude played huge roles in my being successful with the least amount of stress. It is how I choose to see challenges. I am thankful that I am wired that way. I made a promise to myself in August that cancer would not define me. I am more than cancer. I promised myself that I would continue to enjoy each day and slow down or stop when I needed to do so. Additionally, I promised that Frank would not be burdened by my cancer. He needed to be himself and living well. I recognized that I would need help and would accept all support. I think I have lived up to those promises.

I will see my medical oncologist on the 22nd and return to the local hospital for a radiation planning session on the 28th. I have learned that the 16 sessions of radiation are no longer an option because of the chemo. UGH! Now I will have 33 days of radiation. Radiation will be easier to get through. My challenge will be having a daily schedule. I have not had one since I retired.

On Friday, we will celebrate Frank's 54th birthday, the most important day of the year for him. He talks about it daily for 365 days. I look forward to his celebration! He reminded me we need to stretch it out, and we will.

I have not spent lots of "us" time with Frank as I did pre-chemo. We are beginning to capture those important times more frequently. He came downstairs yesterday and said, "Love is the best." Then he made a circle with his arms over his head and told me he loved me to the moon and back. Frank always keeps me centered on what is most important in life. Love him dearly!!

I have a pause between treatment phases. I need a short trip to the beach. Hopefully, I can work out something with my schedule and our caregiver. The beach speaks to my soul. It will reenergize me for the upcoming treatment.

I am pushing to do more and doing well with it. I may have a slow day after a full day, but I can resume full force again. I am walking longer and plan to go more frequently. My goal is to regain my exercise routine of walking five times each week. Exercise always has been the driver of my health. It takes me longer to walk each mile, on the rare days that I can, because of the overall fatigue. I know it will improve in time.

Yesterday I visited a friend whom I have not seen in a few years. Only recently did she hear I had breast cancer. I shared with her my surprise at the support I have received. Friends with whom I have not stayed in close contact jumped in to help immediately. Good friendships remain despite the distance or lack of time. It was the same on this visit. I hope I can do a better job of staying in contact as I regain my health. It is a lesson from this journey. Again, I thank each one of you for your unconditional support of Frank and me. You have lifted me up more than you will ever know.

Enjoy your weekend.

Love,
Marilyn

My friends continue to lift my spirits.

"As ALWAYS your post lifts ME up."

"You go girl".

"You are amazing and have handled this amazingly. — Hope your true energy comes back soon."

I was checking our bank accounts online and noticed a huge error with Frank's health insurance. During my first cycle of chemo in December, I paid his health insurance three times within the same week. I also paid three different amounts. What was I thinking! I guess the chemo was impacting my head more than I realized. I called Anthem, explained my brain fog, asked for forgiveness, and got an update on the account. I made more errors and owed them money. It was an eye-opener for me.

Only now am I realizing the chemo brain is here and has been here for weeks. My thinking is not great. My recall is limited. I intentionally have lived recent weeks in a smaller world to help me get through this journey. As I begin to stretch my thinking again, it is difficult at times. The chemo had a huge impact on my body. I am fatigued but not always aware of how much because of my limited activities. Nothing feels normal anymore.

I drove myself to all four chemo infusions. They were good days. On my compromised days, I stayed home and did what I could. Some days I did nothing. Having chemo put me in a zone. I was aware only of what it was taking to get me through each day. It was a different life, but my life I had to face. I was clueless about how this journey would impact me. I don't think I could have imagined it through someone else's story.

I am glad the chemotherapy treatment is over. Prior to treatment, I had a 15–16% chance of recurrence elsewhere in my body. After treatment, my risk of recurrence was reduced to 10–11%. I certainly want to get any possible reduction, although I wish it could have been reduced more. I do not want cancer again. Let the healing begin! Now I have four weeks to chill before radiation begins.

Radiation Next

I take a short trip to help me regroup and get ready for this next phase. Again, I cannot stress enough the importance of finding time to do something for yourself. It recharges me for the upcoming treatment. This journey continues to test me mentally, physically, and emotionally.

If asked, I would advise anyone to surround yourself with family and friends and welcome the support. Talk to your doctors and let them guide you. Continue enjoying life as best possible under these circumstances. The sun will come up again.

Staying focused on what I need to do daily is significant for me. Eliminating all unnecessary activities and not looking ahead makes it easier.

Radiation Has Begun! — March 14

Dear Friends,

I met with the radiation oncologist and followed it with a planning session. His first comment to me was, "I was shocked that you had chemo." Welcome to the club. No one expected me to have chemo. However, the oddity of my situation with the genetic test tipped the decision. After this planning session, I returned for a recheck of the planning and had X-rays (CT scanner) taken. This process is highly technical. Apparently, more X-rays will be taken weekly. It helps with the computations for my radiation.

The micrometastases in one lymph node will not require radiation. They were treated by the chemo. It means I do not need radiation to any of my lymph nodes. Good news! However, the chemo had little impact on the breasts. Now I am at 30% risk of a recurrence in the breasts without radiation. After radiation, my risk will be reduced to 5%. Recurrence risk elsewhere in my body is 10%–11% after surgery and chemo. I do not pay much attention to the percentages. I was at 3–4% risk of getting breast cancer according to a reminder sent to me. There are no guarantees.
.
Once I began pushing myself all day, I became aware of some forgetfulness. It does not interfere with my overall functioning, but I do know it is happening. Details are not sticking with me. It was evident today when our estate attorney came to see me. Thankfully, she was understanding. The medical oncologist said I will see it improve in the next 2–3 months. The neuropathy continues to be annoying. It can take 6–12 months for it to resolve because these nerves are the farthest away from my body. I find that walking decreases the neuropathy, or it keeps me from thinking about it. I am not sure which part is more accurate. The cells within my body will take more time to heal. Although I am feeling better and more "normal", the chemo symptoms continue to be a part of me. Radiation symptoms will occur later but will heal sooner. Now I

understand more than ever why the breast cancer journey can last for 12–18 months.

I delayed the start of radiation for a few days, so I could spend time at the beach. Frank chose to stay home. He loves his time with Dee. It gave me time to be on the beach, visit with several friends, enjoy seafood, get a massage, and have some downtime. I also put together the frame of a brass bed and got a few small projects done. It is amazing how three nights at the beach can make a huge difference for me. It has been a long seven months since my diagnosis. I came home ready to begin the treatments. My energy has been "restored".

As always, I am intrigued by something new, especially with my health. I am stretched out on the radiation table with my arms overhead and hands reaching for the posts behind me. I must be still. The radiation therapist takes measurements, covers my upper body, and exits the room. A large round machine is above me. I can see plates of steel within it moving back and forth to create different radiation angles. I begin thinking about questions to google and/or ask the oncologist at our weekly meeting. During the radiation, I count to 100 and the machine stops. It moves to my side where I am unable to see it. The radiation begins once more. I only count to 84 this time. The machine stops, and the therapist comes in. She checks positioning and measurements on the other breast, exits the room, and starts the radiation. My count seems less this time. I learn that there is less radiation on one side. It depends on the density of tissue, etc. The overall radiation time is short. It takes 20 minutes from the moment I am called back to the dressing area to the moment I am exiting the building. Sometimes there is a delay in the waiting room. It is why I always carry reading material with me. It prevents unnecessary stress.

I am walking a faster pace now and am excited about it. I am pushing to keep that pace for a longer time. Some walks are 2.5 miles; other walks are 1.5 miles. Two days ago, I walked a sixteen-minute mile. On my worst chemo days, I was walking a 22-minute mile. My physical therapy has made a huge difference in eliminating my movement restrictions. I continue to work on my endurance. Recently, I read that women in their 60s should walk 16-minute miles and walk 10,000 steps daily. I reached 8000 steps recently but have more work to do for consistency. It is obvious that my activity plays a huge part in keeping me healthy.

As I learn more about how long it takes the body to recover from chemo and radiation treatments, I am less concerned with a timeline and more focused on weekly improvement. It is working! I had a tough year from a fall before my diagnosis which compounded the cancer journey. I am healing from the fall and determined to get back in shape again. This goal keeps me focused on something positive while I continue with my treatment.

As of today, I have been treated four times with radiation. I have 29 more treatments ahead of me. Rather than think about getting to the end, I will think about another weekend at the beach midway through the treatments. Those trips keep me balanced.

I am trying to get out more. After my first radiation visit, I drove to Williamsburg and had a shopping spree. I think I deserved it after getting through chemo. Last night I met with a group of friends for dinner. I am looking forward to seeing friends from college this week. On Friday Anna and I will begin walking after my radiation treatments. Life is becoming somewhat normal again!

Thanks again for the continuing support from everyone. Jessica, you truly surprised me today! I have smiled all day!

I hope all of you are enjoying the extended daylight hours. Have a wonderful week!

Love,
Marilyn

Selected comments:

"Wonderful missive as always, Yes, you and Frank have a head strength getting you all through many times when others would give up."

"Marilyn, you are an inspiration. Love you."

"It really sounds like you are doing great. I'm so glad you got to spend some time at the beach recharging. Your description of the actual radiation gave me a real feel for what you are going through. I'll really be thinking about you these next 20+ days and hoping they are without complications. I know you'll be happy to have this behind you and to be moving on to healthier days."

Radiation Update — April 6

Dear Friends,

In my first week of radiation, I attended a "Look Good Feel Better Every Day" class. It is offered by the American Cancer Society at several of our local hospitals. I received a bag loaded with cosmetics and learned how to maximize all of it with the assistance of a cosmetologist. I was motivated to attend in hopes of learning how to compensate for the potential loss of my eyebrows and eyelashes. I now have some strategies if it happens. It was amazing to see the changes in one person who had been struggling and needed a boost.

On day seven I began to experience pink skin and mild burning. Fun times ahead! Because of my fair skin, I am not surprised. From the beginning, I have been putting a cream on my chest three times a day to keep it moist. Now that I am feeling the mild burn, I have added a medicated cream for nighttime. I guess it is the big gun. No creams are allowed during the four hours preceding radiation. Additionally, I must use a deodorant without aluminum. Tom's works well.

My hair is growing slowly. It is soft and feels like hair on a baby. It needs to grow much more before I will let the wig go. I have adjusted to the wig and am enjoying the color and the straight hair. We always want something different from what we have.

Oddly enough, I have hot flashes which only affect my head. I will get a major heat wave rolling through briefly. Months ago, I thought the heat was from wearing a hat all day. Now I realize I was having hot flashes. It can be multiple times a day or none. They seem to be decreasing.

On a different note, Frank came into the kitchen one day and began talking about chemo and my wig. He reminded me that I am "Ms. Kojak". I told him my hair is coming back but it will be a long time before I can give up the wig. He began singing, "How long, how long, oh baby, how long". He said he heard it from a song on Matlock. (true) He does crack me up. Sometimes I find myself wondering how long, how long, oh baby, how long!

My memory is improving. I am thankful! Paperwork and communications got lost at times. If I didn't deal with something immediately, I forgot I needed to get it done. I have increased swelling in my legs on some days. Last Friday I experienced significant swelling in my breasts. I am glad I am not that large daily! The oncologist checks weekly for issues and is helpful in dealing with them. I like how proactive the physicians have been in following me through all treatments. They are a wealth of information.

The oncologist and I discussed basketball games during March Madness. He follows several teams, including the women at Notre Dame. It is fun to work with physicians who are so personable. It makes my visits more enjoyable.

Last week, I completed my 17th treatment. I was at the mid-point. It meant time for me to take a break. Frank and I spent the weekend at the beach and enjoyed our short time there.

One radiation machine has shut down a few times. I had to wait an additional two hours or return later in the day. They had to get someone from Tennessee to fly in and help them after multiple breakdowns. Initially, there was no communication to patients about the delays other than a note taped on the side of the counter when I arrived. It did not give the full picture. I would waste that time and cancel other plans and appointments. We were there for them and at whatever time they got to us. It was not working for me, especially with the frequency of the delays. After conversations with the unit administrator, I now receive calls with a choice to come two hours later or to reschedule later in the day. I also have been given the option to skip that day and add one at the end. I eliminated that option immediately. I want to be done! I have appreciated their receptiveness to my concerns and their working with me on a better plan.

This week, I have an ugly rash on my chest. Hydrocortisone relieves the itching. There is mild discomfort in my entire chest from the cumulative radiation. There is no remedy for the pain which feels like a sunburn. I have some fatigue, but nothing compared to chemo fatigue. I can have full days. These remaining treatments will be interesting. Some patients blister and must take a break. I am hopeful I can stay on schedule and complete treatments as planned.

Compared to chemotherapy, radiation is boring in a good way. I show up, have my treatment, leave quickly, and continue my day. I don't think about it once I leave. Chemo never left my mind. Anna and I are walking immediately after each treatment. It helps to get my walking done before I return home. My endurance has improved. I am getting 10,000 plus steps more often. I am feeling better and better, despite some lingering effects from the chemotherapy. These side effects are receding and are less annoying. I had complete feeling in my feet for three days before the numbness returned to a lesser level. Progress!

21 down, 12 to go! The end of radiation is in sight! I see the light at the end of the tunnel after a long eight months.

Yesterday, I met with the Nurse Practitioner who works with my surgeon. There are no issues. We discussed a follow-up plan. I will have a mammogram in August and an MRI six months later. I will be able to check in with the radiologist to whom I give credit for starting my journey on a positive note, and preventing me from stressing over the diagnosis, and believing that this journey is doable. At the 3-month dates between my imaging, I will see either the medical oncologist or the surgeon. They share responsibilities to reduce the number of medical appointments required. This plan will continue for five years, I think. It is amazing what goes into keeping me healthy. I am blessed to have health insurance and outstanding care. I plan for life to go on and these appointments to be a blip on the screen.

I have decided to take a big trip in the fall to celebrate. I should be recovered fully by then. It is great to think about the months ahead and to look forward to something after only thinking about one day at a time for several months.

Again, thank you for your friendship and prayers, your continuing support throughout my journey, and your willingness to put up with my emails. You continue to be a huge part of my success.

Love,
Marilyn

Some comments:

"Thank you for sharing more about your journey. I feel so blessed to have you to talk to about my situation."
(newly diagnosed lymphoma patient)

"So good to hear your upbeat voice again! I think you have done so well and you are an inspiration! I had a few delays with my radiation also. Keep on the road you are on. A nice trip sounds like a wonderful reward!"

"Great to get such a detailed update, Marilyn. You are doing an amazing job, and I'm so proud of you. I hope we can celebrate with lunch again soon."

"Thanks for your update, Marilyn. We are all looking forward to your last treatment with you. You have had quite a journey. I am impressed with your courage and stamina. I hope you have written our lunch date on your calendar on the 24th."

"WELL, I must say this was a welcome to my FRIDAY. Your positivity and energy in this is unbelievable – well, not really – since it's YOU."

"You're almost there Marilyn!!! Thanks for the update. You are really amazing. I think that so many people will benefit from your being such a great advocate for yourself! I've been thinking of you!"

"Love your continued optimism."

I get blown away by the comments to my emails. I certainly never set out to be inspirational. I simply want to get through it and do what must be done. The many comments, too

I may not have a choice in what happens to me, but I do have choices in how to respond. It takes effort but it's well worth it.

numerous to include, with each email bring me joy, peace, strength, validation, and encouragement. Once again, never underestimate the power of your words to someone going through cancer treatment. These communications serve as a link to the outside world when my world has gotten smaller.

Sometimes I have bumped into obstacles during this journey. We do not live in a perfect world. Errors will be made. It speaks well of a place when the person hears your concerns and take actions to make patient care better. It is another example of the strength of this breast cancer community. They are here for their patients in so many ways.

No More Radiation — April 24

Dear Friends,

The last month brought a load of fatigue, initially on Fridays. By late afternoon, I could barely function. I guess it was the accumulation of radiation during the week. On the other days, I seemed okay. Two weeks later, I realized that my body was slammed with fatigue. I adjusted by having some downtime each day. It did not remove the fatigue but made it easier for me to endure. The fatigue was strong because of the radiation on both sides. I always am surprised when I have a new side effect even though I know it is coming.

I received a text one evening from "your friendly neighborhood dosimetrist" who is the sister of a friend. She did the computer-generated planning for my radiation and invited me to see the design of my treatment plan. I jumped at that opportunity. I love to learn about the details of my treatment. In fact, I have enjoyed the learning that has gone on with this journey. I have found the professionals to be wonderful in helping me understand everything I want to know about my health journey. Believe me, I have asked many questions.

Now I wait for my side effects from all treatments to go away. I continue with a film on my teeth, some loss of sensation in my feet and left lower leg, a slight loss of sensation in my fingers, pain in the bottom of both feet as the numbness begins to recede, hair trying to recover, nails in transition (no polish yet), mild burning in my chest, a red chest with some tightness, swelling in my torso, and only a small amount of fatigue. I imagine the hot weather and strong beach winds will challenge me with this wig. I know Frank will have a role in deciding when I can expose my head again. He does not want "Ms. Kojak's" head to be revealed. At this point, I am getting darker auburn hair with predominately gray hair. I keep reminding myself it will take two cycles of hair growth before I know the final outcome. I will have another adjustment to being me again.

This past weekend, two friends joined me at the beach before my final radiation treatment. It was the beginning of my celebration. My only surprise was a return of the chemo taste when I ate a piece of tart key lime pie yesterday. It has returned my mouth and stomach to a yucky feeling. I find it odd when something will trigger a side effect that I hoped was gone forever. After lingering for a few days, this taste will go away. I will avoid the citrus taste to give my body more healing time.

Today, I received a certificate and rang the bell for completion of radiation and joined friends for lunch at the Urban Farmhouse. Soon, Frank and I will be packing for a beach trip. I can hardly wait to get there and have no schedule. I am returning to my retirement mode.

I have an appointment with the medical oncologist on May 10th. I expect to begin the hormone therapy and hope the medicine will agree with me. There are side effects that may be noticeable. I will see the radiation oncologist on the 25th for a follow up on my treatment.

It has been a long road since August when I was informed by the radiologist that a mass on the ultrasound looked like breast cancer. I remember that visit well. I walked out of the hospital, called Anna, and went home to begin my research, and develop a plan. On August 26th as I was sitting outdoors in Williamsburg, I made a few phone calls and got clarity on an action plan. Today I can proudly say it worked well for me. Thank you, thank you, thank you for your kindnesses, prayers, communications, and loving support throughout my journey with bilateral breast cancer. I have been blessed with an incredible group of supportive friends. The surgery, chemotherapy, and radiation are completed. As I go to the next phase, I feel good about this battle. The hard part is done!

I plan to go off the grid with these group updates. At some point, I will send a follow up when I hope to say I have recovered with side effects gone. I understand some people have a tough time with the transition because of the constant attention throughout many months. No worries here. I will have toes in the sand, a drink in hand, and joy all around. My smile will not stop.

Life has returned to "normal" for us. It only will get better each week. I am embracing the thought of doing more for others and not having to focus so much on me.

Some people see the glass half empty; others see it half full. Some people consider themselves survivors; I choose to consider myself healthy again without the survivor label. There will be no worries about the future. Should cancer rear its ugly head again, I will deal with it. In the meantime, onward with this wonderful life!

Love and hugs,
Marilyn

No more, no more, no more.... DONE!!

Some comments:

> "I read your insights and then think about my mom and all she dealt with. She never shared how she felt. She just took it one day at a time. It would have been helpful to know more about what she was going through. You are an inspiration, just like my mom, about how a positive attitude in adverse situations can bring about favorable results! 38 more days and then I'm free! We need to plan a trip to celebrate both of us!"

> "I'm so happy for you that you are finished and for the process of true healing to begin. What an ordeal only another cancer patient can comprehend. You are an amazingly strong woman."

> "I am so happy for you!! Now get back to retirement!"

> "CONGRATULATIONS!! You did it with panache! So happy the treatment is over. Had a great time starting your celebration this weekend. Hope you keep celebrating a long time."

> "You have been so courageous, so pro-active, so positive and so determined that cancer would not defeat you nor define you. I am proud to be your friend."

> "SO HAPPY FOR YOU! Forward with life! See you around the 'hood, my friend!!!"

> 'So happy this part is behind you!"

It is strange reading these comments and to hear that friends believe I have been so strong. That word is not one I thought about during treatment. It was more survival and trying to get through it the best way possible. I am convinced my positive outlook on life, in general, played a huge part in this journey.

Recovery

May 9

I have my post-chemo visit with the medical oncologist tomorrow. In reviewing my notes, I plan to discuss the leg swelling, numbness in my hands and feet, and breast pain on the sides of both surgeries. It is evident that the side effects of chemo and radiation will continue. My underarms are beginning to become tight. It makes a full range of motion difficult without considerable pain. I see progress overall!

May 10

I always enjoy my visits with this oncologist. She is personable, caring, and always has time for discussion. Her physical exam checks everything from neck to waist. I like the comprehensiveness of looking for possible indications of more cancer. She starts me on letrozole for the next five years. Like chemo, it is a global treatment. Side effects may occur over time with possible hair thinning, joint pain, and stiffness. The hair thinning does not concern me because my hair is unusually thick, more so than prior to chemo. Joint stiffness may challenge me since I deal with it now. I was fortunate not to lose either my brows or lashes.

June
I experienced some shortness of breath from the radiation.
It only lasted a week, thankfully. I knew it might occur but
was surprised.

Rarely do I experience side effects from medications. However, the letrozole challenged me during the first week. I have
been on it for a month now and never notice any side effects.
Because of the potential for bone thinning, I will have a bone
scan during the next year.

July
My underarms are tight, tight, and tight. I am assuming it
occurred during the radiation boost over those last few days.
The angle of the machine was changed. The last five days of
radiation are called a boost. The radiation focuses solely on the
tumor sites. It is going to take work and time to release this
tightness. I only notice it when I stretch my arms in any direction. When they are by my side, I do not have any discomfort.

August 9
I met with the medical oncologist today. I asked if I am cured
or dealing with a chronic disease. Since there is a risk of cancer
returning, I am not cured. It is the bad part of cancer. There
always is a chance it will show up again. We discussed the neuropathy. I no longer have it in my hands. With my feet, most
often I feel numbness in my toes. The breast pain is milder.
It was caused by the radiation. I have experienced hot flashes
throughout this past year. Now I seldom have them. I hope it
stays that way. They were not always easy to get through.

August 10
I return for my first mammogram after treatment. It is normal. I will follow it with an MRI in six months because of
the denseness of my breasts and bilateral breast cancer. The
best part of this visit is having a few minutes to reconnect
with my wonderful radiologist. I continue to credit her with
the calmness of my year with cancer. I continue to believe
my learning about breast cancer enhanced my conversations
with my physicians and made for a stronger experience.

Creating a plan for how to get through this journey was significant for me. Never have I gone through anything serious so calmly. I honestly have no regrets and do not know how I could have done it differently to get the desired outcomes.

No More Cancer! — August 10

Dear Friends,

It has been one year since my diagnosis. My mammogram today was normal. My visit with the medical oncologist yesterday was positive. I have no signs of cancer! Amen! Because I do have a risk of the cancer returning, I am in remission and not cured. I obviously will never rid myself of this cancer label. Yet, I can push it to the back of my mind and not give it any attention. I also have been discharged by the radiation oncologist. For follow up, I will be seen every three months. I am celebrating!

The summer months have allowed much healing. My first pedicure in months was a bit challenging. My feet are overly sensitive. The bottoms of the feet remain painful, but I am glad to feel again. The numbness most often is confined to the area around the toes but can return to the entire foot with more activity. I have a few more months to get my feet back to normal.

My hair remains crazy curly. It looks like I had a permanent. The auburn color is beginning to overpower the gray. The oncologist thinks my hair will return to my original look by the end of the year. I will get my hair trimmed tomorrow for the first time since December. Chemo kills cancer cells but leaves so much damage to the body. I easily see why it is an 18-month journey when chemo is part of treatment.

Frank has gotten comfortable with the words "cancer" and "chemo". He says he hears Andy Griffith say it on Matlock. Thank goodness, I have Andy with Frank! The hair is a different issue. He has struggled with it for months. At the beach in July, I told him it was time for me to stop wearing a hat and being myself. My hair was short and looked different. It does not seem to be stressful for him now. He transitioned well and rarely comments on it.

To celebrate my getting through this breast cancer journey, I am going with a dear friend to Hawaii for two weeks in October. Hawaii is one of three states I have not visited. We will stop for a couple of days in San Francisco to break up the trip. I am excited. Frank will stay home. He is equally excited about having Dee here with him. It is a win-win for both of us!

There will be no more group updates about my journey unless cancer rears its ugly head again. I thank each of you for every kindness extended to me and/or Frank. Looking back, I know now I was not aware of how much this journey took out of me. I am blessed to have wide support from our friends who truly made sure I was taken care of during some difficult months. Without you, my story would be quite different. I am grateful for these friendships and all you did.

Hugs and love,
Marilyn

Selected comments:

"What wonderful news!!! I know the year has been beyond painful, literally and figuratively, but you kicked c's butt. I applaud you celebrating in tangible ways. Just enjoy the curls."

"Just reading this, Marilyn, with tears in my eyes, and joy and gratitude in my heart. What a blessing. But, oh, what a journey for you, and for Frank. Let's try to have lunch next week if you are free. Thanks for allowing me to travel this journey with you. I am more thankful and grateful than ever before."

"What a beautiful story to end the week! So grateful to God and the Universe for allowing the end of your journey to be so positive and appreciative."

"I am joining you with many praises for God's care and guidance on this journey! Happy vacation celebrating to you and Frank! Love you, Lady!"

"I have tears of joy and thanksgiving for you!! I am thrilled with this wonderful news, and I know you are, too. You have been an amazing and inspiring role model for all of us, and I so admire how you've handled the illness, your approach and attitude, and Frank and his feeling about all of this. Your celebration plans to visit Hawaii sound wonderful, and I know that will be such a good time for you. Well deserved, my friend!!"

"Woohoo, and thanks be to God! So glad to hear this news. Love and hugs."

"Is it me, or does it seem we have lived about 3 years in 1! So happy this is behind you and so proud of your brave journey. Thank you for allowing me to travel with you as you have moved toward a cancer-free life."

"WHOOPPEEE! You have fought hard and you are seeing the pay off! Your positiveness has helped so many! God is good and has watched over you and Frank."

"Such a positive and welcome letter! You are dear to our family and we rejoice when you do! I am glad you are going to Hawaii. Sounds like a winner!"

"This is fantastic news and I am so happy for you. What a journey and from what I can tell one that you have navigated bravely and fiercely."

"Praise God! I am thrilled for you! Enjoy a much-deserved vacation in Hawaii!"

October 5
I had an appointment with my surgeon. No concerns were noted in her examination of my breasts. I had an opportunity to ask questions. I am scheduled to return to her office in six months to see the nurse practitioner. They alternate the six-month visits. I plan to see a gynecologist in the same month and hope she will assume the responsibility for the cancer check. Then I can drop one appointment. It is time to streamline my appointments where appropriate.

With each month passing, my hair continues to make changes. It remains thicker than ever. I have some visible gray and certainly have more curl. It looks good after some months of looking in the mirror and wondering who I am. There are many stages of hair growth after chemo. It began looking like my auburn color and then was totally gray once I had a full head of hair. It gradually returned to my auburn color. Frank struggled with my looking different for several months. He now sees I am looking more like myself. Our hair stylist has been tremendous with her support. She has been accurate throughout the year in telling me what to expect each month when I take Frank for his haircut. I have some chemo hair which indicates the changes are not finished. It generally takes two complete cycles of hair growth to return to a person's original hair.

To celebrate my battle with breast cancer, I took a two-week vacation to Hawaii. We visited three islands and loved every day of our trip. It was great to go to new places and try to move beyond this past year. I truly enjoyed Kauai, snorkeling, and our helicopter tour of the Napali coast. We built in time to be still and soak in the air around us.

November 22
The neuropathy created challenges for me throughout the year. It slowly receded. The last couple of months, it remained mostly in my toes. I had some days without noticing it and others with it returning full force. It certainly has its own timetable. The pain and/or numbness in my feet has been annoying. It has taken much longer than I expected to restore normalcy.

The tightness with my underarms is minimal. I have a full range of motion without difficulties. I have no hair growth with my underarms and no longer perspire there. The radiation oncologist expected it to return soon after radiation but no luck.

December 30
To my surprise, I had many flashbacks of my time in chemo as I went through this month. I love the Christmas season and had a far different one during treatment. Last year, the Christmas season was challenging. I know it was equally difficult for Frank. I think it took getting healthy again before I could reflect on where I had been to get to this point. I am realizing more and more how weak I was during those treatment months. At the time, I only focused on one day at a time and rarely looked beyond that day. I am proud of my health journey to treat breast cancer. I certainly did not want cancer of any kind. I believe I met the challenges as best I could by listening, learning, tapping into the wealth of knowledge with the physicians, restricting my daily schedule, walking, eating well, continuing to enjoy life, and having terrific support from friends. Best of all was having Frank, my loving brother, by my side. I know he struggled and hurt when I was in treatment. He suffered by watching me. In recent months we have spent time reinforcing the need to heal. I think we have made it! I am hoping the waters will be calm regarding my health in this new year. Life is good and what we choose to make it.

January 17
I met with the medical oncologist. She is referring me to an oncology neurologist for my symptoms which seem like neuropathy again. My feet are numb, and the soles burn. I use a walking pole to neutralize my balance concerns. I am doing well overall and receive a positive report. I had no stress going into this visit. I always expect the best and look forward to having time to chat.

February 4
It has been 18 months since my initial diagnosis and nearly a year since treatment with breast cancer. I will have a breast

MRI, recommended by the radiologist, as a follow up to my mammogram last August. These results will give me stronger confirmation that I am free of breast cancer. Since an MRI discovered one of my tumors, I want this follow up. It will give me an extra dose of confidence that all is well within my body.

I am in a good place emotionally, physically, and mentally. My hair is coarse with curls and darker than before. It is thick and does not feel like my old hair. I can live with it. It is amazing that my body can return to "normal" after absorbing the poison of chemo. I continue with some issues in my feet. I am hoping it will resolve with more time. It remains to be seen.

February 8
My extraordinary radiologist sent a text that my MRI results are normal. It is wonderful news!! This report gives me the confidence to close the book on the medical part of cancer. It brings me full circle with the radiologist whom I respect to the highest degree. I value her expertise and feel better than ever now. I will continue with checkups every three months for the next two years. Then I will graduate to every four months for the following three years. I have enjoyed the new friendships from this journey and imagine I will see other avenues for volunteer work as others face breast cancer.

I received this statement in an email from the radiologist in a response to a comment from me. "I am happy to hear your body is healing some, although the journey will be hard to put behind you no matter how well you do medically." Wow, what a statement and my reality! I so hoped I could close the book on cancer. I guess I was in denial. I wanted to be done with it. I realize now it will never happen. I see differently now and pay attention to anything and everything to do with cancer. It is on my radar screen. I have a keen interest and a greater understanding of what people endure in their battles with cancer. I never think about the possibility of it returning. I can't worry about what I will be unable to control.

I continue to have problems with my feet and issues with my balance and gait from chemo. It is noticeable and does get in my way. My hair remains thick and somewhat curly. It feels like my hair now. Otherwise, I have returned to my life without cancer. So thankful!

April 15
Thankfully, I no longer think about cancer every day. However, it is woven into me now and will always be a part of who I am. I have learned, grown, and appreciated so much from this experience.

May 2
I have an answer to the lingering problems with my feet! Neuropathy was ruled out. Chemo neuropathy does not return. Once I get in bed at night, my feet no longer have the issues. I awaken with my feet feeling good. Once my feet are placed on the floor, the symptoms start again. With neuropathy, I had symptoms 24/7. An EMG showed I had no response to the lateral and medial nerves in my feet. The neurologist said it was not concerning. It was due to old age. I was not willing to accept this general diagnosis. I went home, googled this information, and consistently found sites on tarsal tunnel syndrome.

I have been diagnosed with tarsal tunnel syndrome (very rare), plantar fasciitis, and Achilles tendinitis by an orthopedist. I developed a different gait because of balance issues during

I continue to believe that my advocating proactively for my health is key to my successful recovery.

chemo. This different gait compressed the nerves in the tarsal tunnels in both ankles. This compression caused the pain and numbness impacting my balance. It was an entrapment issue. This physician explained that the nerves have short circuits and are unable to function properly. I am relieved to have an explanation and a plan for treatment. It may take six months for the nerves to heal.

August 23
I am well enough that I was able to enjoy outdoor experiences at Glacier National Park and Waterton-Glacier International Peace Park. Time to celebrate again and enjoy more adventures during my retirement!

As I complete my story, I continue receiving physical therapy to restore my feet to good health. I can see the light at the end of this LONG road. I am working to strengthen my ankles for the stability needed with my gait. Obviously, it has taken longer than anticipated for my overall recovery.

I look back over the past two years and am relieved to be at this point. I am cancer free. I remain grateful for new friendships, the breast cancer medical community, and our friends. My care has been outstanding.

Lessons Learned

1. This journey is a family journey. Helping my family and friends understand what I was experiencing provided more support for me in return.

2. Identifying physicians who would be good matches for me was significant. I trusted them and relied on them to problem solve as issues appeared. The relationships are deeper within this extraordinary medical community.

3. Creating a plan for how to get through this journey and sticking to it were huge contributors to my health. Never have I gone through any medical crisis so well. Never have I experienced anything close to this experience.

4. Learning as much as possible about my diagnosis helped me converse with my physicians and kept me from being overly stressed. Yes, I thought about cancer every day, but it was not the stress of fear. It was most often the stress of changes in my body during chemo treatment and adjusting to changes that were unimaginable to me.

5. Every kindness received made a tremendous difference in keeping me positive and moving forward. Friends from college, work, the neighborhood, travel, and church appeared without being asked. I was amazed to see friends I had not seen in years. Once a good friend, always a good friend, regardless of the direction life takes us! I hope to pay more attention to sharing kindness to others in need.

6. There is a huge community of professionals and volunteers to support breast cancer patients throughout this long journey. I tried to be open to the many avenues of support and chose what would be best for me. Everyone's journey is different. Everyone must create their own path based on what will work for them.

7. If something seemed wrong during my treatments, I addressed the issue with the professionals. I always found them to be good listeners and focused on what was best for me. They readily made changes to what needed to be done. This approach minimized additional stress for me.

8. Taking a few short trips away from home was healing. It reinforced my belief in trying to keep a balance during crisis as well as during good times.

9. Breast cancer treatment has become more personalized. Medicine continues to evolve with ongoing research. New findings may change management in the future for patients.

Acknowledgments

A special thank you to Nicole, my phenomenal radiologist, for reviewing the drafts, fact checking the medical information, and encouraging me during this lengthy writing process.

Thank you to Beth Ayn for reading an early draft of my story and helping me see how it could teach others to advocate and be positive in their journeys. Thank you to Kathy, Anna, Rosemary, and Pat for reading drafts and providing helpful feedback.

Thank you to Shirley for editing my story for errors I may have missed.

Thank you to Ben, my graphic designer, for guiding me and taking me step by step to get my story published. You are awesome!

Once you have read this story
and are done, please consider
passing it on to someone
who might benefit.

Made in the USA
Las Vegas, NV
27 January 2025